Enhancing Primary Care Delivery - Systems, Communities, and Clinical Practice

Edited by Thomas R. Wojda

Published in London, United Kingdom

Enhancing Primary Care Delivery - Systems, Communities, and Clinical Practice
http://dx.doi.org/10.5772/intechopen.1008604
Edited by Thomas R. Wojda

Contributors
Ahmed Ali Al-Mohammed, Bethany Fenton, Brahim Zaadoud, Brianna Clark, Craig Field, Darcelle Schouw, Darcy McCampbell, Daryl O. Traylor, Devki Patel, Eboni E. Anderson, Emmanuel Ohakpougwu, Hamad Rashid Al Mudahka, Irene Ramavhoya Thifhelimbilu, Ishaaq Datay, Kgothatso Nkoana, Meghan Etsey, Melitah Rasweswe Molatelo, Michael Mncedisi Willie, Michalina Piechocka, Musa Gumede, Naomi Levitt, Nayla Cheema, Noora Alkaabi, Percy Daames, Peter Delobelle, Phakamile Nkomo, Przemysław Śpiewak, Saad Shahbal, Samantha Iyaloo, Selby Masekela, Steve Reid, Takalani Edith Mutshatshi, Tumelo Assegaai, Youness Chbab

First published in London, United Kingdom, 2026 by IntechOpen
IntechOpen is the global imprint of INTECHOPEN LIMITED, registered in England and Wales, registration number: 11086078, 167-169 Great Portland Street, London, W1W 5PF, United Kingdom

For EU product safety concerns: IN TECH d.o.o., Prolaz Marije Krucifikse Kozulić 3, 51000 Rijeka, Croatia, info@intechopen.com or visit our website at intechopen.com.

British Library Cataloguing-in-Publication Data
A catalogue record for this book is available from the British Library

Enhancing Primary Care Delivery - Systems, Communities, and Clinical Practice
Edited by Thomas R. Wojda
p. cm.
Print ISBN 978-1-83635-376-8
Online ISBN 978-1-83635-375-1
eBook (PDF) ISBN 978-1-83635-377-5

If disposing of this product, please recycle the paper responsibly.

Meet the editor

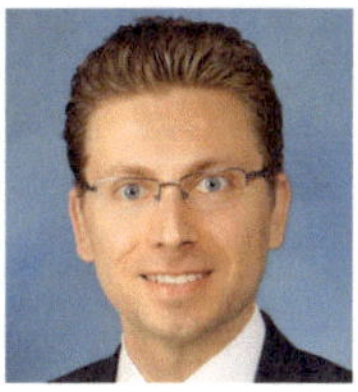

Thomas R. Wojda, MD, MBA, CAQSM, FAIM, is a board-certified Family and Sports Medicine physician and a Clinical Informaticist at the University of Pittsburgh Medical Center, where he currently practices primary care while serving as a physician informaticist in Central Pennsylvania. He received his medical degree from the Medical University of Warsaw, completed primary care residency training at St. Luke's University Health Network, and fellowship training in Sports Medicine at Conemaugh Memorial Medical Center. He completed a Clinical Informatics Fellowship at the University of Pittsburgh in 2025. His work focuses on clinical workflow optimization, digital health, and health system improvement. Dr. Wojda has authored more than 50 peer-reviewed publications, including book chapters and edited volumes.

Contents

Preface

Primary care remains the foundation of effective, equitable, and sustainable health systems worldwide. However, how primary care is organized, delivered, measured, and experienced continues to evolve in response to demographic change, rising non-communicable disease burden, workforce constraints, and increasing system complexity. *Enhancing Primary Care Delivery – Systems, Communities, and Clinical Practice* brings together diverse perspectives that examine how primary care is being re-imagined across settings, populations, and health systems, with particular attention to prevention, integration, quality, and practical implementation.

The volume opens with *Hospital-Based Preventive Medicine Model: Primary Care in a Tertiary Setting*, which explores the integration of preventive and primary care services within hospital environments. This chapter examines how tertiary care settings can serve as platforms for comprehensive prevention and chronic disease management, highlighting opportunities and challenges inherent in hospital-based primary care models. Complementing this systems-level perspective, *Innovative Service Delivery in Primary Health Care: Evaluating Unjani Clinics, Retail Health, and Public-Private Partnerships* examines alternative models of care delivery, focusing on access, financing, and essential benefits within evolving primary care ecosystems.

Attention then turns to prevention and population-oriented care in *Non-communicable Disease Prevention and Care in Community Oriented Primary Care (COPC): Lessons from South Africa*, which illustrates how community-oriented primary care frameworks can be leveraged to address chronic disease through participatory and community-based approaches. This theme is further extended in *Ward-Based Community Healthcare Workers' Challenges Regarding the Utilization of Non-communicable Diseases Screening Tools, Limpopo Province, South Africa*, which highlights frontline challenges faced by community healthcare workers and underscores the importance of implementation support for effective screening and prevention strategies.

The lived experience of healthcare delivery during periods of disruption is addressed in *The Impact of COVID-19 on Primary Health Care-Seeking Behaviour: Voices of Learner Nurses from a Selected University in Limpopo Province, South Africa*. Through the perspectives of learner nurses, this chapter offers insight into how crises influence health-seeking behavior, training environments, and perceptions of primary care access and trust.

Measurement and accountability are central to strengthening primary care systems. *Measuring Performance Quality in Health Care: Relevance and Validity of the Frameworks* provides a critical examination of quality measurement frameworks, discussing their applicability, limitations, and relevance to primary healthcare settings. This chapter offers a conceptual foundation for aligning quality indicators with the realities of frontline care delivery.

Care coordination and integration are explored in *Practical Care Coordination for Primary Care Providers: Bridging the Gap between Clinical Practice and Patient Outcomes*, which focuses on interprofessional collaboration, health information management, and social determinants of health. The chapter emphasizes practical strategies that enable primary care teams to navigate fragmented systems and improve patient outcomes.

The volume concludes with chapters centered on clinical reasoning and the therapeutic relationship. *Motivational Interview Applications for Aiding Therapeutic Alliance in the Era of Social Media Misinformation: An Integrative Review* examines how motivational interviewing techniques can support patient engagement and trust in an increasingly complex information environment. Finally, *Perspective Chapter: Management of a Patient Complaining of Vertigo or Dizziness in General Practice* provides a pragmatic, case-oriented approach to a common yet diagnostically challenging presentation in primary care, illustrating the continued importance of clinical judgment and coordination with specialty care.

Together, these chapters reflect the multifaceted nature of modern primary care delivery. By bringing together system-level models, community-based approaches, quality frameworks, coordination strategies, and clinical perspectives, this edited volume aims to provide readers with a practical, globally relevant understanding of how primary care can be strengthened to meet contemporary health challenges.

The editor would like to thank the contributing authors for their scholarly engagement and commitment to advancing primary care delivery, as well as the editorial and production teams whose efforts supported the development of this volume.

Thomas R. Wojda
University of Pittsburgh Medical Center,
Mechanicsburg, Pennsylvania

Section 1

Models of Primary Care Delivery and System Integration

Chapter 1

Hospital-Based Preventive Medicine Model: Primary Care in a Tertiary Setting

Noora Alkaabi, Ahmed Ali Al-Mohammed, Saad Shahbal and Hamad Rashid Al Mudahka

Abstract

Healthcare systems are increasingly overwhelmed by the global rise in non-communicable diseases (NCDs), with hospitals primarily designed for reactive care and advanced disease management. This model, coupled with rising patient complexity, has created a critical gap in preventive services, leaving early intervention and risk reduction underutilized within hospital settings. This chapter presents a transformative model that reimagines the role of tertiary hospitals, not merely as centers for advanced disease management, but as proactive hubs for preventive medicine. By integrating primary care principles into specialist hospital systems, the model aims to bridge the longstanding divide between prevention and intervention, shifting institutional focus toward long-term health promotion, risk reduction, and continuity of care. The chapter also details the conceptual foundation, structural components, implementation process, outcomes, and policy recommendations of a hospital-based preventive medicine model piloted at Hamad Medical Corporation (HMC) in Qatar. The HMC experience demonstrates how preventive health services, including comprehensive screening, lifestyle counseling, and multidisciplinary collaboration can be successfully embedded into tertiary care settings. This integration not only improves access and continuity of care but also realigns health system priorities toward person-centered, sustainable models of care delivery. By offering a practical framework and strategic insights, this chapter supports the broader adoption of hospital-based prevention models, illustrating their potential to reduce disease burden, enhance health system efficiency, and promote equity across populations.

Keywords: preventive medicine, tertiary care, primary care integration, hospital-based model, lifestyle intervention, non-communicable diseases

1. Introduction

Preventive medicine in hospital-based care refers to a strategic approach that emphasizes risk identification, lifestyle modification, and early detection of disease within the hospital setting itself [1]. Unlike traditional prevention confined to primary care or community outreach, hospital-based preventive medicine capitalizes on every clinical encounter, whether inpatient or outpatient, as an opportunity to screen, counsel, and engage patients in long-term wellness. Integrating primary care principles into tertiary hospital workflows ensures continuity, coordination, and person-centeredness, especially for patients with complex or chronic conditions. This model strengthens care transitions and reduces reliance on fragmented, episodic care that characterizes many tertiary systems.

Hospital-based preventive services align with global objectives of Universal Health Coverage (UHC) and the World Health Organization's (WHO) call for health systems to shift from reactive care to anticipatory, population-health strategies [2]. Major urban centers and networks like the Strong Cities initiative advocate for integrated hospital-community models, recognizing that large hospitals in metropolitan areas are uniquely positioned to scale equitable preventive care [3].

In Qatar, where diabetes, obesity, and sedentary lifestyles are prevalent, embedding prevention within hospitals has become a strategic necessity. An internal wellness assessment in 2024 at Hamad Medical Corporation (HMC) found that 27% of staff were obese, 13% smoked, and physical activity levels were below recommended thresholds. These findings catalyzed the launch of the hospital's preventive medicine mission.

2. Background and rationale

Hospital systems around the world are increasingly challenged by fragmented care pathways, often resulting in disjointed service delivery, redundant procedures, and gaps in follow-up, especially for patients with chronic conditions [4]. Tertiary care hospitals, while equipped with advanced diagnostics and specialist services, tend to operate as siloed departments with limited integration of preventive strategies [4]. This structure hampers holistic, continuous care and fails to capitalize on critical patient encounters to intervene earlier.

Meanwhile, non-communicable diseases (NCDs) are now the leading cause of death globally, accounting for over 70% of all mortality [5]. Conditions like cardiovascular disease, diabetes, chronic respiratory disease, and cancer are not only preventable in many cases but also highly manageable with early intervention. However, in tertiary hospital settings, care is typically initiated only after symptoms become severe or complications emerge. For example, data from the Global Burden of Disease Study indicates that late-stage presentations of NCDs are linked to both increased healthcare costs and higher rates of disability-adjusted life years (DALYs) [6].

This misalignment between where care is delivered and when it is most effective demands a paradigm shift. Hospitals must move from reactive to proactive care models, embedding screening, counseling, and risk stratification into their core services [7]. Encapsulating preventive medicine within hospital walls can reduce admissions, enhance patient satisfaction, and support long-term system sustainability [8].

3. Methods

3.1 Study design

A mixed-methods design was selected, combining both quantitative and qualitative approaches to provide a comprehensive understanding of the hospital-based preventive medicine model. The project was implemented in a tertiary hospital—Hamad Medical

Corporation in Qatar. The implementation was phased over a period of 12 months for pre-launch and initial stage, with more phases rolling out in future as the service expands with additional collaborations.

3.2 Participants

Participants in this phase primarily included hospital staff and high-risk outpatient groups such as geriatric and pediatric populations. For employees, inclusion criteria encompassed all staff categories—clinical and administrative—at HMC, as well as geriatric and pediatric patients attending specialty outpatient clinics.

3.3 Data collection methods

Data were collected through various methods such as internal assessments through data reviews and questionnaires, in addition to the qualitative data captured during the clinical visits. The validity and reliability of the utilized tools were ensured through pilot testing and expert review. Quantitative data included biometric measurements, while qualitative data was gathered through structured interviews focusing on quality of life and overall health.

3.4 Intervention

The intervention during the initial stage involved initiation and integration of preventive health services into routine hospital workflows. This included cardiovascular risk screening, lifestyle assessments, smoking cessation programs, and weight management counseling. The intervention was implemented using a multidisciplinary approach comprising preventive medicine physicians, clinical dietitians, health educators, psychologists, and nursing staff.

3.5 Data analysis

Quantitative data was analyzed using statistical software, with descriptive and inferential statistics employed to identify trends and associations. Qualitative data was analyzed thematically, with coding and categorization performed to identify key themes and patterns.

4. The HMC model of hospital-based preventive medicine

Hamad Medical Corporation, being the largest tertiary healthcare provider in Qatar, recognized the urgent need to address the rising burden of NCDs within its own clinical environment. In response, the Preventive Medicine Division was established to integrate preventive health services into existing hospital workflows, transforming routine clinical encounters into opportunities for risk assessment, early intervention, and patient empowerment.

4.1 Target population and clinical setting

The model was initially launched in late 2023 with a focus on HMC's internal staff across all job categories, including clinical and administrative employees.

This decision leveraged the workplace as a controlled environment ideal for piloting preventive strategies, with staff acting as both beneficiaries and champions of change.

The model soon expanded to include high-risk outpatient groups, notably geriatrics and pediatric patients attending specialty clinics. Plans are underway to offer these services to broader patient groups through inpatient and outpatient departments and executive health clinics.

4.2 Clinical services offered

Preventive care is embedded within routine care pathways and delivered through dedicated hospital-based preventive medicine clinics. Services are offered as either standalone consultations or integrated within regular specialist appointments. Key services include the following:

- Cardiovascular risk screening: Regular monitoring of blood pressure, fasting glucose, lipid profiles, and HbA1c to identify individuals at elevated risk for atherosclerotic disease or diabetes [9].

- Comprehensive lifestyle assessment: Structured interviews and questionnaires assess diet quality, physical activity, sleep hygiene, and stress levels informing personalized lifestyle intervention plans.

- Cancer screening: Evidence-based screening is provided for breast and colorectal cancer risk assessment aligned with national guidelines [10].

- Smoking cessation: Behavioral counseling and pharmacotherapy options are made available through structured tobacco cessation clinics, with follow-up integrated into EMRs [11].

- Weight management and physical activity counseling: Patients receive guidance tailored to their readiness for change, supported by group education, motivational interviewing, and mobile health tools [12, 13].

These services are aligned with Qatar's National Health Strategy priorities, including reducing the burden of chronic disease and enhancing wellness promotion [14].

4.3 Role of the multidisciplinary team

A defining characteristic of the HMC model is its emphasis on multidisciplinary collaboration. Preventive care is delivered through a coordinated team that includes preventive medicine physicians who oversee patient evaluation, screening, and clinical decision-making lifestyle and behavior intervention. They also lead case discussions and program refinement. Additionally, clinical dietitians provide tailored nutrition plans, particularly for patients with metabolic risk or obesity, while health educators deliver health literacy materials, facilitate workshops, and guide behavior change using structured models like the transtheoretical mmmmodel. Th team also includes psychologists and behavioral therapists to help address underlying mental health challenges, readiness to change, and coping strategies. Nursing Staff support in conducting screenings, providing brief interventions, and assist in patient navigation.

The administrative team includes administrative and data officers who track population outcomes, monitor electronic medical records (EMR) prompts, and generate dashboards to support quality improvement.

This collaborative framework ensures that each patient receives individualized care, while contributing to population-level improvements in health outcomes [15, 16].

5. Implementation strategy

Implementing a hospital-based preventive medicine model at HMC required a phased, structured approach to ensure successful integration across clinical settings, sustained engagement from health professionals, and alignment with institutional goals. The strategy emphasized streamlined workflows, embedded use of health IT systems, and patient-centered education.

5.1 Implementation phases and activities

This phased model ensured adaptability, stakeholder ownership, and measurable improvements in early detection and lifestyle risk reduction. **Table 1** elaborates on the implementation phases of the PM model at HMC.

5.2 Patient flow and referral systems

A centralized Preventive Medicine Team coordinated follow-ups, maintained referral logs, and liaised with primary care or specialist clinics to ensure longitudinal care continuity. Preventive consultations were integrated into patient care in two primary formats:

- *Embedded consults*: For patients attending specialty outpatient clinics (e.g., Cardiology), preventive assessments were added as part of their scheduled visit using structured EMR prompts.

- *Standalone appointments*: For high-risk individuals or those requiring follow-up, dedicated preventive medicine consults were booked independently, allowing more time for counseling and multidisciplinary interventions.

Phase	Activity	Description
Phase 1	Design	Development of standardized clinical protocols, screening algorithms, EMR documentation templates (via Cerner), and staff training modules. This phase also included the creation of referral pathways, Standard Operating Procedures (SOPs), and Key Performance Indicators (KPIs) aligned with national standards.
Phase 2	Pilot	Preventive services were first piloted at the Staff Medical Center. The focus was on hospital employees, providing cardiovascular risk screening, lifestyle assessments, weight management, cancer risk assessment, mental health screening and tobacco cessation. The pilot helped refine workflows, test EMR integration, and gather user feedback.
Phase 3	Scale-Up	Services extended to departments including Cardiology, Oncology, Endocrinology, Executive Health Clinics, and Geriatric and Pediatric services. Co-located preventive consultations were introduced alongside regular specialty visits. Preventive metrics were embedded into routine clinical audits.

Table 1.
Implementation phases and activities of HMC PM model.

Referral pathways were established with internal departments (e.g., nutrition, psychology, smoking cessation clinics). Referrals were facilitated using Cerner-based templates that ensured uniform data entry and triggered necessary workflows.

5.3 EMR integration (Cerner)

Cerner played a pivotal role in integrating preventive workflows into routine care delivery. Smart alerts flagged eligible patients based on age, diagnosis codes, and missed screenings (e.g., mammogram overdue). Decision support tools prompted clinicians to address risk factors like smoking, obesity, or prediabetes during visits and structured templates were used to capture lifestyle behaviors (diet, exercise, and stress), readiness to change, and follow-up planning. KPI dashboards monitored real-time clinician compliance (e.g., BMI documentation, counseling rates) and fed into department-level performance reviews. This integration of standardized delivery reduced missed opportunities for prevention and improved clinical accountability.

5.4 Health promotion campaigns and education

Multiple initiatives like public awareness campaigns and outreach activities helped increase preventive health literacy, drive patient engagement, and normalize prevention as a routine part of hospital care. A robust patient and staff education framework supported clinical delivery.

- Awareness campaigns: Aligned with national and international health days (e.g., Breast Cancer Awareness Month, World Hypertension Day), these campaigns featured activity booths, educational talks, and staff wellness drives.

- Multilingual resources: Culturally tailored brochures, digital QR-code flyers, and video content were produced in Arabic, English, and other major languages spoken by staff and patients.

- Onsite counseling: Health educators and dietitians were stationed in outpatient clinics and waiting areas to provide counseling and brief interventions.

- Professional development: CME-accredited workshops and e-learning modules trained clinicians on behavior change communication, motivational interviewing, and preventive care guidelines.

6. Tools and technology

The integration of digital infrastructure is essential to the effective implementation and scalability of hospital-based preventive medicine. At HMC, technology has been strategically leveraged to support screening, risk identification, workflow optimization, and data-driven decision-making. The following components represent core digital enablers in the HMC model.

6.1 EMR integration and clinical decision support

The Cerner EMR system was customized to support preventive workflows. Algorithms embedded within Cerner automatically flag patients eligible for screenings based on age, gender, chronic disease profile, and risk factors. These automated cues improved clinician adherence to national preventive care protocols and streamlined documentation during busy outpatient visits.

For example:

- Breast cancer screening alerts were generated for women aged 45–69 who had no recent mammogram documented.
- Colorectal cancer screening reminders were issued for patients aged 50–74.
- Tobacco users, patients with elevated BMI, and those with prediabetes or poorly controlled hypertension triggered decision support prompts for lifestyle counseling, nutrition referral, or smoking cessation.

6.2 Digital health tools for patient engagement

Research indicates that digital tools can significantly improve health behavior adherence and promote sustained lifestyle change when paired with provider feedback and reinforcement [17, 18]. HMC piloted several digital engagement tools to enhance patient participation in preventive care:

- Mobile apps and web-based portals allowed patients to self-monitor lifestyle indicators such as daily physical activity, weight, blood pressure, and dietary patterns.
- Personalized health reminders were generated based on the patient's risk profile and EMR data, nudging them to schedule follow-ups or complete health education modules.
- Some applications included gamified interfaces and goal-setting features, which boosted engagement, especially among younger patients and tech-savvy populations.

6.3 Dashboards and analytics

Real-time data dashboards were developed for use by clinicians, department leads, and hospital administrators to help in monitoring real-time quality data [19]. The dashboards were reviewed monthly as part of departmental quality meetings. In one example, low documentation of physical activity counseling in cardiology clinics led to a targeted CME training session and EMR template revisions. These dashboards served three primary functions:

- *Population risk surveillance*: Visualizations of trends in obesity, smoking prevalence, HbA1c levels, and screening compliance across departments or sites.
- *Clinician performance monitoring*: Dashboards displayed preventive KPI compliance for individual providers or units (e.g., percentage of eligible patients screened, smoking status documented).
- *Service utilization tracking*: Enabled tracking of preventive consult volumes, patient no-show rates, and referral completion.

6.4 Interoperability and future integration

Efforts are underway to further enhance interoperability between Cerner and digitized mobile platforms, enabling real-time data exchange, personalized health notifications, and patient-generated data incorporation into clinical care plans. This aligns with the digital health component of Qatar's national health strategy and offers future opportunities for integrating predictive analytics and machine learning algorithms to identify high-risk patients in real time and tailor interventions more precisely.

7. Evaluation and outcomes

Evaluating the effectiveness of a hospital-based preventive medicine model is essential to validate its impact, ensure continuous improvement, and guide scalability across institutions. At HMC, a combination of clinical metrics, operational indicators, and patient-centered outcomes was used to measure program success.

7.1 Clinical outcomes

- *Improved screening rates*:
    - o Colorectal cancer screening and risk assessment uptake increased from 42–70% among eligible staff and patients within the first 18 months of implementation.
    - o Breast cancer risk assessment and screening compliance rose by 22%, supported by Cerner alert prompts and coordinated follow-up systems.
- *Chronic disease risk reduction*:
    - o Among participants enrolled in preventive services, the average BMI decreased by 1.9 kg/m^2 per month.
    - o Mean HbA1c levels dropped by 0.5% among individuals with prediabetes who received counseling and follow-up.
    - o Over 28% of tobacco users referred to cessation clinics reported sustained abstinence for 6 months or longer.

7.2 Operational metrics

- *Utilization trends*:
    - o Preventive service visits in the staff medical center and HMC geriatric clinic (geriatric wellness services) and pediatric clinic (pediatric preventive medicine services) increased by 85% after the program launch.
    - o More than 83% of eligible patients had complete documentation of lifestyle risks (e.g., smoking status, BMI, and physical activity) in the EMR.

- *Provider engagement*:
  - Departments demonstrated a 78% average compliance with preventive KPIs, aided by dashboard feedback loops and performance incentives.
  - Overall, preventive medicine clinicians completed CME-accredited training in lifestyle counseling and motivational interviewing.

7.3 Patient-centered indicators

- *Satisfaction and engagement*:
  - Patient satisfaction with preventive care consultations improved from 76–95%, as measured by post-visit surveys.
  - Over 1200 patients accessed QR-linked digital health flyers in Arabic and English, indicating growing digital engagement.
- *Continuity of care*:
  - Integrated care plans and follow-up alerts in the EMR improved appointment adherence by 19% and reduced redundant referrals.

7.4 Institutional impact

- *Policy uptake*:
  - The success of the pilot led to formal inclusion of preventive services in departmental scorecards and strategic planning documents.
  - The model informed institutional quality improvement (QI) projects, particularly in staff wellness and chronic disease screening.

8. Challenges and lessons learned

Implementing a hospital-based preventive medicine model in a tertiary care setting—Hamad Medical Corporation—presented several operational, cultural, and systemic challenges. These obstacles provided key insights that helped refine the model over time.

8.1 Challenges

8.1.1 Clinician resistance to workflow changes

Despite the strong clinical rationale, initial resistance was perceived among few healthcare providers accustomed to traditional, reactive models of care. Concerns included increased consultation time, unclear roles in preventive counseling, and skepticism regarding the effectiveness of lifestyle interventions in acute care environments. These attitudes are not unique to HMC and have been documented in similar hospital-based initiatives elsewhere, particularly where behavior change is seen as outside the remit of specialist care [20–22].

8.1.2 Limited awareness of preventive medicine among staff

A baseline needs assessment at HMC revealed that many clinical and non-clinical staff had limited understanding of preventive medicine principles. Misconceptions included equating prevention solely with vaccination or health education, rather than a structured, multidisciplinary approach embedded in clinical workflows.

8.1.3 Logistical constraints and scheduling barriers

Coordinating multidisciplinary services, securing space within existing outpatient clinics, and integrating preventive consultations into busy tertiary schedules posed significant logistical hurdles, risking burnout among the healthcare workers [23]. Additionally, referral pathways varied by department, which complicated standardization and timely service delivery.

8.1.4 Inconsistent documentation and KPI monitoring

Early phases of the project highlighted inconsistent documentation of preventive measures in the EMR. For example, smoking status and physical activity levels were often left blank or recorded in free text, limiting auditability and performance tracking.

8.2 Lessons learned

8.2.1 Leadership endorsement and policy alignment were crucial

Top-down support from hospital executives and departmental heads significantly accelerated program adoption. Formalizing preventive services into institutional strategic plans and quality improvement (QI) targets fostered accountability and ownership.

8.2.2 Training and success stories built staff engagement

CME-accredited workshops on motivational interviewing, EMR usage, and chronic disease counseling improved staff confidence. Sharing early success stories, such as weight loss milestones or reduced HbA1c levels, helped generate buy-in across departments and illustrated tangible patient benefits.

8.2.3 Clear KPIs and performance dashboards motivated participation

Visual dashboards displaying screening rates, BMI documentation, and smoking cessation referrals were introduced as part of the institutional quality framework. Departments with high performance were recognized, reinforcing a culture of competition and excellence in prevention.

8.2.4 Flexibility and iterative feedback were essential

Pilot programs were used as feedback loops. Adjustments to EMR templates, referral forms, and educational content were made based on user feedback, ensuring the program remained adaptive to clinical realities.

9. Discussion: A paradigm shift

The implementation of a hospital-based preventive medicine model at Hamad Medical Corporation (HMC) marks a significant shift in how tertiary institutions contribute to health promotion and disease prevention. Traditionally, tertiary hospitals have been positioned at the end of the healthcare continuum, focused largely on managing complex, late-stage illnesses. However, with non-communicable diseases (NCDs) accounting for over 75% of global mortality, healthcare systems are increasingly recognizing the necessity of shifting upstream to intercept disease earlier in the care pathway [24].

9.1 Comparison with global models

Globally, a number of health systems have piloted similar integrations of prevention into hospital settings, particularly in response to the rising burden of lifestyle-related diseases. In the United States, the Kaiser Permanente system has demonstrated success in embedding preventive screenings and chronic disease management into its hospital and outpatient workflows, leading to significant reductions in hospitalization rates and costs [25]. In Singapore, hospitals under the National University Health System (NUHS) have adopted population health strategies, including risk stratification and hospital-based wellness clinics, targeting high-risk individuals even before the onset of disease [26].

Closer to the region, initiatives in Saudi Arabia's Ministry of Health hospitals have incorporated structured screening programs for diabetes and hypertension at the point of hospital entry, resulting in improved case detection and referral rates [27].

Compared to these models, HMC's approach is uniquely positioned in that it combines:

- Integration into existing clinical services, not requiring separate vertical programs;
- Robust EMR-supported workflows using Cerner to automate risk alerts and decision support;
- Multidisciplinary teams operating across specialties (e.g., endocrinology, cardiology, family medicine); and
- Simultaneous implementation of community-facing health promotion campaigns.

These features allow for both clinical depth and population reach, enabling HMC to bridge hospital care with public health functions.

HMC's experience illustrates that with structured workflows, executive leadership, and digital infrastructure, even complex tertiary hospitals can play a central role in improving population health outcomes. The successful implementation of preventive medicine within a tertiary hospital in Qatar provides a replicable model for health systems globally, particularly those in high-income or rapidly developing countries experiencing dual burdens of chronic disease and rising healthcare costs.

10. Policy and strategic recommendations

To scale the hospital-based preventive medicine model effectively, strategic policy actions are required at both the institutional and national levels. The success of the implementation at Hamad Medical Corporation (HMC) underscores the importance of leadership, infrastructure, and sustained commitment to prevention. The following recommendations are drawn from HMC's experience and global best practices.

10.1 Embed preventive KPIs into accreditation and performance reviews

Regulatory bodies and hospital accreditation frameworks should embed preventive medicine indicators into their evaluation criteria. These could include the following:

- Percentage of eligible patients screened for cancer or chronic disease risks
- Documentation of lifestyle risk factors (BMI, smoking status, and activity level)
- Clinician compliance with brief intervention protocols

Integrating these KPIs into performance appraisals, department dashboards, and pay-for-performance models reinforces accountability and institutional prioritization of prevention [28].

10.2 Allocate funding for preventive staff and digital tools

A preventive model cannot function without adequate human resources and technological support. Policy planners and hospital administrators must understand the long-term benefit of investing in:

- Preventive medicine physicians and allied health professionals (e.g., dietitians, health educators, and psychologists)
- IT infrastructure including EMR integration, dashboards, and decision support systems
- Digital engagement tools (e.g., patient portals and mobile apps)

Cost-effectiveness studies suggest that investments in preventive infrastructure yield long-term savings by reducing admissions and complications from unmanaged NCDs [29, 30].

10.3 Institutionalize preventive medicine departments within hospitals

Hospitals should formally establish dedicated preventive medicine units or integrate preventive functions into core departmental structures. This institutional presence ensures that prevention is not treated as an auxiliary service but rather as an essential clinical function. These departments can oversee screening initiatives, lead staff training, and collaborate with specialty clinics to embed preventive protocols into routine care pathways. As seen in other systems, such as Kaiser Permanente and NUHS Singapore, institutional alignment enhances scalability and quality assurance [25, 26, 31].

10.4 Promote research on hospital-based prevention

Despite growing interest, hospital-based prevention remains under-researched and under-appreciated globally. National funding agencies, hospital research divisions, and academic institutions should support implementation science, cost-effectiveness analysis, and patient outcome studies related to tertiary-based preventive care [32–34]. At HMC, the integration of real-world data analytics and EMR-based tracking allows for continuous quality improvement and research publication, thus contributing to the global evidence base.

11. Future directions

The hospital-based preventive medicine model at Hamad Medical Corporation (HMC) marks a pivotal shift in how tertiary care institutions can champion early intervention and long-term wellness. To sustain this progress and scale its impact, future development should focus on strategic system expansion, deeper community integration, capacity building, and data innovation.

11.1 Full expansion to tertiary sites

Building on the successful pilot programs, HMC is poised to expand preventive services across all tertiary hospitals and specialty clinics. This includes embedding lifestyle and risk factor screening into oncology, cardiology, endocrinology, geriatrics, and pediatric services. Standardized clinical pathways, EMR integration, and co-located consultations will support this scale-up and ensure continuity of care across all departments. The long-term vision is to integrate prevention as a routine part of every hospital visit.

11.2 Strengthened hospital-community linkage

To enhance population health outcomes, hospitals must extend their reach beyond facility walls. Future efforts will emphasize formal referral loops to primary care, partnerships with community health centers, and outreach campaigns to promote early community engagement. Lessons from integrated systems like the WHO's Health in All Policies approach [35] and "accountable communities for health" in the U.S. [36] demonstrate that bridging hospital-community divides is essential to closing prevention gaps.

11.3 Enhanced training pipeline

Sustainable delivery of preventive services requires a skilled workforce. HMC plans to expand clinical fellowship and residency training in preventive medicine, while also embedding lifestyle counseling and health promotion modules in undergraduate and nursing education [37, 38]. Continued Medical Education offerings focused on motivational interviewing, digital health engagement, and chronic disease prevention will support ongoing staff development across specialties [31].

11.4 Use of predictive analytics

The next frontier in hospital-based prevention lies in harnessing predictive analytics and artificial intelligence (AI) to personalize risk management. HMC aims to enhance its EMR-based algorithms using real-world data and machine learning models to stratify patients based on modifiable risk factors, social determinants, and genomic profiles. Such tools can prioritize high-risk patients for targeted intervention, improving outcomes and optimizing resource allocation [39, 40].

12. Conclusion

The hospital-based preventive medicine model introduced at Hamad Medical Corporation demonstrates that tertiary care institutions have substantial potential to evolve from reactive treatment centers to proactive hubs for health promotion, early detection, and chronic disease prevention by integrating primary care principles into hospital workflows. The approach capitalizes on the existing infrastructure of tertiary hospitals while reconfiguring service delivery to prioritize upstream interventions. The model's clinical and operational feasibility can be ascertained through the benefits observed such as improved cancer screening rates, reductions in cardiometabolic risk factors, increased provider engagement, and enhanced patient satisfaction.

Looking ahead, there is significant potential to scale this model across Qatar's broader health system and adapt it internationally. Strengthening hospital-community linkages, leveraging predictive analytics, and embedding preventive competencies in clinical training pipelines will contribute to overall improvement in population health outcomes and quality of life. With institutional commitment, digital innovation, and inter-sectoral collaboration, hospital-based prevention can become a cornerstone of universal health coverage and long-term health system resilience.

Acknowledgements

The authors acknowledge the leadership of the Hamad Medical Corporation and Corporate Department of Medicine, the Preventive Medicine Division team, and all participating clinicians and staff who contributed to the design, implementation, and evaluation of this model. The authors acknowledge the use of Microsoft Copilot (AI tool) for language polishing of the manuscript.

Conflict of interest

The authors declare no conflict of interest.

Author details

Noora Alkaabi[1,2]*, Ahmed Ali Al-Mohammed[3], Saad Shahbal[3]
and Hamad Rashid Al Mudahka[4]

1 Preventive Medicine Division, Department of Medicine, Hamad Medical Corporation, Qatar

2 QU Health, Qatar University, Qatar

3 Department of Medicine, Hamad Medical Corporation, Qatar

4 Preventive Medicine, Primary Health Care Corporation, Qatar

*Address all correspondence to: nalkaabi@hamad.qa

References

[1] Rodrigues da Silva AC, Sousa da Silva KG, Torres Costa T, et al. The importance of preventive medicine in reducing chronic diseases. Environmental and Social Management Journal / Revista de Gestão Social e Ambiental. 2024;**18**(2):1-11. DOI: 10.24857/rgsa.v18n2-040

[2] World Health Organization. Universal Health Coverage (UHC). 2023. Available from: https://www.who.int/news-room/fact-sheets/detail/universal-health-coverage-(uhc)

[3] Urban Institute. 1st Annual Report White House Council on Strong Cities, Strong Communities. In Urban Institute; 2013. Available from: https://www.urban.org/sites/default/files/2018/05/31/sc2_1st_annual_report.pdf

[4] Europe WHORO for, Policies EO on HS and, Nolte E, Pitchforth E. What is the evidence on the economic impacts of integrated care? iriswhoint. 2014;11. Available from: https://iris.who.int/handle/10665/332002

[5] World Health Organization. Noncommunicable diseases: key facts; 2023. Available from: https://www.who.int/news-room/fact-sheets/detail/noncommunicable-diseases

[6] Vos T, Lim SS, Abbafati C, et al. Global burden of 369 diseases and injuries in 204 countries and territories, 1990-2019: A systematic analysis for the global burden of disease study 2019. Lancet. 2020;**396**(10258):1204-1222

[7] Alley DE, Asomugha CN, Conway PH, et al. Accountable health communities—Addressing social needs through Medicare and Medicaid. The New England Journal of Medicine. 2016;**374**:8-11

[8] Sofia Razzakh S, Singh R, Uddin Khan B, Hassan N. The health-promoting lifestyle behaviors of healthcare employees in Qatar - A cross-sectional comparative study. 2024;**Qatar Medical Journal, 2024**(4):74. DOI: 10.5339/qmj.2024.74

[9] World Health Organization. HEARTS: Technical Package for Cardiovascular Disease Management in Primary Health Care: Risk-based CVD Management. www.who.int. Published July 13, 2020. Available from: https://www.who.int/publications/i/item/9789240001367

[10] Ministry of Public Health. Cancer Clinical Guidelines. Available from: https://www.moph.gov.qa/english/departments/healthaffairs/NCDPP/nationalcancerprogram/cancerclinicalguidelines/Pages/default.aspx.Weill Cornell Medicine-Qatar. Certificate in Lifestyle Medicine. https://qatar-weill.cornell.edu/event/certificate-in-lifestyle-medicine; 2019

[11] Ministry of Public Health. Tobacco control; 2017. Available from: https://www.moph.gov.qa/english/strategies/Supporting-Strategies-and-Frameworks/QatarPublicHealthStrategy/Pages/Tobacco-control.aspx

[12] Ministry of Public Health. National Clinical Guidelines: The Diagnosis & Management of Obesity in Adults. 2024. Available from: https://www.moph.gov.qa/_layouts/download.aspx?SourceUrl=/Admin/Lists/ClinicalGuidelinesAttachments/Attachments/197/The%20Diagnosis%20and%20Management%20of%20Obesity%20in%20Adults.pdf

[13] Aspetar. Qatar National Physical Activity Guidelines 2nd Ed; 2021.

Available from: https://www.aspetar.com/AspetarFILEUPLOAD/UploadCenter/637736948034432931_QATAR%20NATIONAL%20PHYSICAL%20ACTIVITY%20GUIDELINES_ENGLISH.pdf

[14] Ministry of Public Health. National Health Strategy 2024-2030; 2024. Available from: https://www.moph.gov.qa/english/NHS/Pages/Priorities.aspx

[15] Prochaska JO, Velicer WF. The transtheoretical model of health behavior change. American Journal of Health Promotion. 1997;**12**(1):38-48

[16] Frieden TR. A framework for public health action: The health impact pyramid. American Journal of Public Health. 2010;**100**(4):590-595

[17] Kayser L, Kushniruk A, Osborne RH, Norgaard O, Turner P. Enhancing the effectiveness of consumer-focused health information technology systems through eHealth literacy: A framework for understanding users' needs. JMIR Human Factors. 2015;**2**(1):e9. Published 2015 May 20. DOI: 10.2196/humanfactors.3696

[18] Fadahunsi KP, Akinlua JT, Oke J, et al. Information quality frameworks for digital health technologies: Systematic review. Journal of Medical Internet Research. 2021;**23**(6):e23479

[19] Twohig PA, Rivington JR, Gunzler D, Daprano J, Margolius D. Clinician dashboard views and improvement in preventative health outcome measures: A retrospective analysis. BMC Health Services Research. 2019;**19**(1):475. Published 2019 Jul 11. DOI: 10.1186/s12913-019-4327-3

[20] Brull R, Ghali WA, Quan H. Missed opportunities for prevention in general internal medicine. CMAJ. 1999;**160**(8):1137-1140

[21] Khoja Q, Algarm Z, Alsuwailem S, Alrumaihi S, Alqahtani T. Knowledge, attitude, and prevalence of lifestyle medicine practice among family physicians in primary care centers in Saudi Arabia. South Eastern European Journal of Public Health. 2025;**16**(1):1926-1938. Available from: https://www.seejph.com/index.php/seejph/article/view/4046

[22] Abdulrahman AAAA. Knowledge and attitude of lifestyle medicine-based approach among health care providers working in Dubai academic and health corporation. World Family Medicine. 2024;**22**(7):14-23

[23] Bodenheimer T, Sinsky C. From triple to quadruple aim: Care of the patient requires care of the provider. Annals of Family Medicine. 2014;**12**(6):573-576

[24] World Health Organization. Noncommunicable Diseases: Key Facts. World Health Organization; 2025. Available from: https://www.who.int/news-room/fact-sheets/detail/noncommunicable-diseases

[25] McCarthy D, Mueller K. Kaiser Permanente: Bridging the Quality Divide with Integrated Practice, Group Accountability, and Health Information Technology; 2009. Available from: https://www.commonwealthfund.org/publications/case-study/2009/jun/kaiser-permanente-bridging-quality-divide-integrated-practice

[26] Pushing Frontiers. Future-Proofing our People: Advancing a population's Health and Development. Singapore: Nanyang Technological University; 2025. Available from: https://www.ntu.edu.sg/research/research-hub/news/detail/future-proofing-our-people--advancing-a-population's-health-and-development

[27] Alarifi AM, Alshahrani NZ, Jokhdar H, Asiri AM. Advancing health through sustainable development goals-Saudi Arabia's mid-journey progress and insights. Journal of Epidemiology and Global Health. 2025;**15**(1):48

[28] Kruk ME, Gage AD, Arsenault C, et al. High-quality health systems in the sustainable development goals era. The Lancet Global Health. 2018;**6**(11):e1196-e1252

[29] Berwick DM, Nolan TW, Whittington J. The triple aim: Care, health, and cost. Health Affairs (Millwood). 2008;**27**(3):759-769

[30] Bodenheimer T. Coordinating care—A perilous journey through the health care system. The New England Journal of Medicine. 2008;**358**:1064-1071

[31] Vallis M, Lee-Baggley D, Sampalli T, et al. Equipping providers with principles, knowledge and skills to successfully integrate behaviour change counselling into practice: A primary healthcare framework. Public Health. 2018;**154**:70-78

[32] Gold MR, Realmuto L, Scherer M, Kamler A, Weiss L. Community priorities for hospital-based prevention initiatives: Results from a deliberating public. Journal of Public Health Management and Practice. 2018;**24**(4):318-325

[33] Cowie J, Nicoll A, Dimova ED, Campbell P, Duncan EA. The barriers and facilitators influencing the sustainability of hospital-based interventions: A systematic review. BMC Health Services Research. 2020;**20**(1):588. Published 2020 Jun 28

[34] Rechel B, Durvy B, Augusto GF, et al. Primary prevention in hospitals in 20 high-income countries in Europe—A case of not "making every contact count"? Health Policy. 2025;**151**:105199

[35] WHO. Promoting Health in All Policies and intersectoral action capacities. World Health Organization. Published 2018. Available from: https://www.who.int/activities/promoting-health-in-all-policies-and-intersectoral-action-capacities

[36] Prevention Institute, JSI Research and Training Institute, Inc. Accountable Communities for Health A "Portfolio of Strategies" Approach to Improving Population Health. Published February 2016. Available from: https://www.preventioninstitute.org/publications/accountable-communities-health-portfolio-strategies-improving-community-health

[37] Chong SCS, Anderson K, Mackenzie-Stewart R, Hobbs C, Conna B. Embedding experiential learning in undergraduate health promotion curriculum. Health Promotion Journal of Australia. 2022;**33 Suppl 1**(Suppl 1):9-16

[38] Modena G, Mazzoleni B, Sponton A, et al. Nursing students' perceptions of barriers, facilitators and solutions in their role as health promoters: Findings from a qualitative study. Nursing Reports. 2025;**15**(7):232

[39] Obermeyer Z, Emanuel EJ. Predicting the future - big data, machine learning, and clinical medicine. The New England Journal of Medicine. 2016;**375**(13):1216-1219

[40] Topol EJ. High-performance medicine: The convergence of human and artificial intelligence. Nature Medicine. 2019;**25**(1):44-56

Chapter 2

Innovative Service Delivery in Primary Health Care: Evaluating Unjani Clinics, Retail Health, and Public-Private Partnerships

Michael Mncedisi Willie, Samantha Iyaloo, Kgothatso Nkoana, Phakamile Nkomo, Selby Masekela, Percy Daames and Musa Gumede

Abstract

This study investigates the contributions of private-sector innovations to strengthening primary health care (PHC) in South Africa through a systematic literature review. Grounded in the health systems strengthening framework and the primary health care approach, the review critically analyses key private initiatives, including nurse-led Unjani Clinics, retail pharmacy-based health services, and public-private partnerships (PPPs). These models demonstrate significant potential in improving accessibility, scalability, and efficient resource use within the PHC system, particularly in underserved urban and rural communities. The findings highlight how private-sector involvement can complement public health efforts by extending service reach, empowering frontline health workers, and optimising limited health resources. Despite these positive contributions, the study identifies equity, policy coherence, and long-term sustainability challenges. Private-sector models sometimes risk exacerbating health disparities if not fully aligned with universal health coverage goals and national health strategies. Moreover, the sustainability of PPPs and retail services depends heavily on regulatory oversight, clear quality standards, and robust governance frameworks. To maximise the impact of private-sector participation, the study recommends enhanced policy integration, strengthened collaboration between public and private actors, and rigorous monitoring to ensure alignment with South Africa's national health priorities and the overarching principles of equity and social justice in PHC delivery.

Keywords: primary health care, private sector, health systems strengthening, Unjani clinics, public-private partnerships, retail health services, South Africa, universal health coverage

1. Introduction

Stark inequities between the public and private sectors mark South Africa's healthcare system. While the private sector serves just under 15% of the population, it consumes a disproportionately high share of national health expenditure and possesses significantly more resources and healthcare professionals [1, 2]. South Africa's health system reforms have advanced towards universal health coverage, yet persistent inequalities and human resource shortages demand coordinated, rights-based, and community-driven interventions to ensure quality, equity, and resilience [3]. Most of the population depends on the overstretched public health system, where access to quality primary health care (PHC) is often compromised by staffing shortages, infrastructure challenges, and limited service availability [4, 5]. Strengthening PHC is critical to achieving universal health coverage (UHC) and reducing the burden on higher levels of care [4, 6].

Globally, PHC is recognised as a key driver of equitable and cost-effective health systems. The World Health Organisation (WHO) underscores PHC as the cornerstone for strengthening health systems, particularly in low- and middle-income countries. It emphasises its centrality in achieving universal health coverage and advancing the Sustainable Development Goals (SDGs) [7]. Strengthening primary health care is the most cost-effective way for low- and middle-income countries to achieve universal health coverage and improve health outcomes, particularly for marginalised populations [8]. A key finding from the WHO [9] states that scaling up PHC interventions in low- and middle-income countries could save 60 million lives and increase average life expectancy by 3.7 years by 2030. In South Africa, primary health care re-engineering is a central focus of the National Health Insurance policy reform, highlighting the need for strengthened partnerships between the public and private sectors to address workforce shortages and improve the equitable distribution of healthcare professionals, supported by aligned Human Resources for Health strategies to enhance implementation success [10]. This chapter explores the gaps in PHC provision in South Africa and examines the contributions and lessons from the private health sector in addressing these gaps. Drawing on case studies and emerging models of care, it highlights how private initiatives have improved access, quality, and efficiency in PHC delivery.

2. Literature review

2.1 Gaps in primary health care delivery

The foundational role of PHC in achieving UHC is well-documented globally [11]. PHC improves population health outcomes by delivering integrated, accessible, and person-centred services near where people live and work [12]. In South Africa, the public sector has historically borne the primary responsibility for PHC delivery. Numerous studies have underscored persistent systemic challenges across both public and private healthcare systems. Within the public sector, issues such as chronic underfunding, inadequate infrastructure, human resource constraints, and fragmented service delivery have significantly impeded the effectiveness of PHC [13, 14]. In contrast, the private sector's limited benefit coverage for PHC further restricts its accessibility and effectiveness, with allocations declining to less than 6% of total benefits paid [2]. These parallel challenges across the public and private sectors highlight the urgency for coordinated reform, aligning with the objectives of PHC re-engineering under the National Health Insurance (NHI), which aims to transform service delivery by fostering greater collaboration, innovation, and integration across the health system.

Scholars increasingly argue for a more integrated approach, where the strengths of both sectors are harnessed to build a resilient health system [15, 16]. Achieving UHC requires effectively integrating targeted health interventions into existing health systems through a systems-thinking approach, supported by a pragmatic balance of public-private participation, and strong government stewardship to ensure sustainability and good governance [15, 17]. Strengthening PHC systems in low- and middle-income countries through standardised performance measurement and shared best practices can enhance care quality, accessibility, and effectiveness [18]. In pursuing a more equitable and inclusive health system, South Africa must move towards a unified approach, transcending public-private divides. Effective collaboration could include shared service delivery models, integrated training platforms, and interoperable health information systems. Achieving this vision requires intentional policy alignment, robust accountability mechanisms, and incentive structures that prioritise quality care and equity over profit-driven imperatives, commonly associated with the private sector [19–21]. The literature emphasises that meaningful integration requires more than rhetorical commitment: it necessitates deliberate efforts to build trust, establish shared governance structures, and promote active community engagement. In the absence of these measures, South Africa may continue to reinforce a dual health system that disproportionately benefits a minority, while compromising equitable access for the broader population.

2.2 Innovations and partnerships in strengthening PHC delivery

A notable case study illustrating efforts to reprioritise PHC through shared goals is the South African private innovative Unjani Clinic network. This nurse-led initiative, from refurbished shipping containers, has significantly enhanced access to PHC services, especially in underserved and rural communities [22]. These clinics provide low-cost, accessible PHC services to communities that often fall outside the reach of the public health system. With over two hundred operational sites nationwide, Unjani Clinics is a scalable model for community-based care that empowers nurses as frontline providers, while expanding the geographic footprint of healthcare delivery [22]. Retail health services have also played an increasingly significant role in PHC delivery. Chain pharmacies, such as Clicks and Dis-Chem, have incorporated in-store clinics, offering various services, including immunisations, health screenings, and basic consultations [23, 24]. These models are perceived to reduce the burden on public clinics and improve convenience for working individuals and families in urban and peri-urban areas. However, the commercial orientation of such models often raises concerns about affordability and equitable access for low-income groups, especially when these pharmacies are not nearby.

Public–private partnerships (PPPs), collaborative arrangements between government entities and private sector organisations for the delivery of public services have demonstrated substantial potential in closing critical service delivery gaps, particularly in regions experiencing acute shortages of public healthcare personnel [25, 26]. For example, initiatives that deploy private practitioners to rural hospitals to deliver maternal and obstetric care have effectively alleviated human resource constraints while improving service quality. However, the success of such public-private health collaborations hinges on robust government stewardship, enhanced regulatory capacity, and strategic alignment with national health priorities. Furthermore, systematic monitoring and evaluation are essential to scaling up these partnerships sustainably and mitigating potential unintended consequences [25]. Despite these evident benefits, persistent challenges remain regarding regulatory oversight, quality assurance, and coherence with broader national health objectives. This underscores the pressing need for a more integrated and coherent policy framework to ensure private-sector innovations are scalable and contribute equitably and sustainably to the national PHC agenda. Without such integration, PPPs risk fragmenting the health system and undermining efforts towards universal health coverage.

3. Theoretical framework

This study is underpinned by the health systems strengthening (HSS) framework and the PHC approach, as articulated by the WHO [27] and Witter et al. [28]. The HSS framework identifies six core building blocks of an effective health system: service delivery, health workforce, information systems, medical products and technologies, health financing, and leadership/governance [29]. These elements ensure equitable, quality, and sustainable health care. This framework helps analyse the private sector's role in reinforcing public health functions, particularly in under-resourced and under-served communities. The PHC approach, rooted in the Alma-Ata [30] and Astana [31] Declarations, and emphasised by Kraef and Kallestrup [32], promotes comprehensive, community-centred care as essential to UHC. The figure below illustrates how strengthening PHC, reaffirmed as a global priority 40 years later, advances SDG 3 by supporting universal coverage, health security, and related targets, highlighting the need for combined public and private sector contributions, as depicted in **Figure 1** below.

This figure illustrates how HSS, through core pillars, such as infrastructure, workforce, financing, and governance, can advance Sustainable Development Goal 3 (SDG 3) when grounded in PHC principles and a strong public health orientation. PHC foundations emphasise community-based, person-centred, and accessible

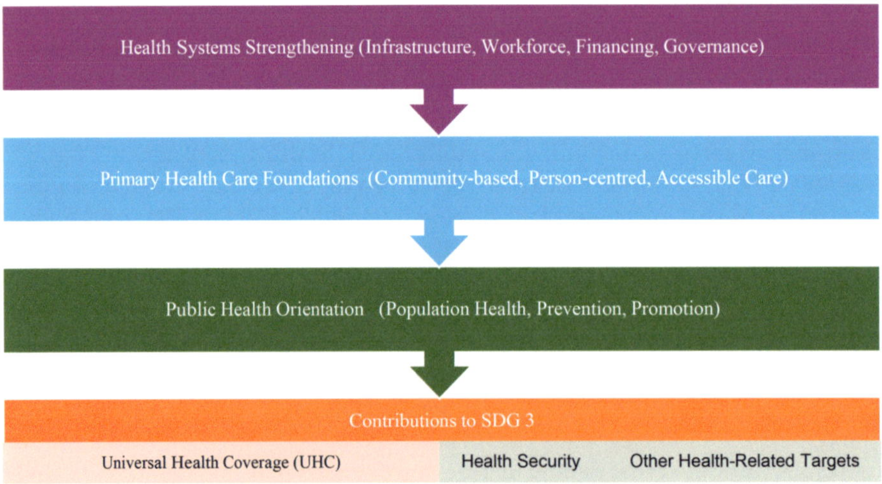

Figure 1.
Health Systems Strengthening Framework. Source: Adapted and expanded from WHO [27], Witter et al. [28], and Kraef and Kallestrup [32].

services, while a public health approach prioritises prevention, promotion, and population-level interventions. Together, these components drive progress towards UHC, enhanced health security, and other health-related targets. This study critically examines how private sector innovations such as Unjani Clinics, retail pharmacies, and public-private partnerships (PPPs) contribute to or deviate from these goals, with specific attention to issues of equity and access [22]. Institutional theory as an analytical lens evaluates how regulatory frameworks, policy environments, and socio-economic forces influence their integration and effectiveness in advancing public health outcomes [32].

4. Research methods

This study adopts a literature review methodology to explore the role of private sector innovations in strengthening South Africa's PHC system. A literature review is appropriate given the study's objective of synthesising existing knowledge, identifying conceptual gaps, and drawing policy-relevant lessons from diverse private-sector interventions [33]. It enables the critical engagement with empirical findings, policy reports, and theoretical debates across multiple disciplines, including public health, health systems research, and development studies [34, 35].

A structured search was conducted across reputable academic databases. It was supplemented by grey literature from policy institutions such as the Health Systems Trust, the South African Department of Health, and the WHO. Keywords used in the search included *primary health care*, *private sector health*, *public-private partnerships*, *Unjani Clinics*, *retail health services in South Africa*, and *health systems strengthening*. To ensure relevance and currency, the search included peer-reviewed journal articles, government policy documents, and organisational reports published between 2010 and 2024 [34, 35]. Inclusion criteria required that sources be.

- focused on South Africa or offered regional or global insights applicable to the South African context,
- engaged substantively with PHC or private sector contributions, and
- presented empirical findings, policy analysis, or conceptual frameworks. Studies not available in English or lacking sufficient methodological transparency were excluded from the review [33].

The selected literature was subjected to thematic analysis to identify recurring patterns, contradictions, and insights about private-sector contributions to PHC. The study was structured around the WHO HSS framework, enabling a systematic assessment of how private innovations contribute to key health system components such as service delivery, workforce development, and governance. Particular attention was paid to how lessons from models such as Unjani Clinics, retail pharmacy services, and PPPs align with PHC values of accessibility, equity, and community participation [22]. Themes were analysed deductively and inductively using established health systems theory, allowing new insights to emerge from the literature. This approach ensured both conceptual rigour and sensitivity to context-specific dynamics.

A structured search was conducted across multiple academic databases, including **MEDLINE**, **Scopus** and **Web of Science**, covering literature published between

2010 and 2024. The search was complemented by grey literature from key policy and health organisations such as the South African Department of Health (2021), the Health Systems Trust (2023), and the WHO (2020). Keywords included combinations of *primary health care*, *private sector health*, *public-private partnerships*, *Unjani Clinics*, *retail health services in South Africa*, and *health systems strengthening*.

Sources were included if they:

- Focused on South Africa or provided regional/global insights relevant to the South African context.
- Substantively addressed PHC or private sector contributions.
- Presented empirical findings, conceptual frameworks, or policy analyses [25].

Sources were excluded if they:

- Were not available in English; or
- Lacked sufficient methodological detail or transparency.

A total of 47 sources were included in the review, comprising peer-reviewed journal articles (61.7%), grey literature (12.8%), policy documents (8.5%), working papers (6.4%), books (4.3%), and case studies (6.4%). As summarised in **Table 1**, this mix of source types ensures academic depth and practical relevance. Notably, **70.2%** of the sources were published between **2018 and 2025**, reflecting the most recent developments in PHC, private sector engagement, and health system reform.

Source type	Number of sources	Year range
Peer-reviewed journal articles	29	2005–2025
Grey literature/reports	6	2021–2024
Books/book chapters	2	2014–2016
Working papers/scoping protocols	3	2023–2025
Policy documents/declarations	4	1978–2018
Case studies/conceptual models	3	2016–2021

Table 1.
Overview of included sources by type and year range.

5. Results

5.1 Scalable and sustainable service delivery models

The review found compelling evidence that nurse-led innovations, particularly the Unjani Clinics model, provide scalable and sustainable solutions to gaps in PHC coverage. The Unjani Clinics model demonstrates a strategic integration of nurse empowerment, holistic care, innovative financing, and tailored technology, as summarised in **Table 2**. This multifaceted approach addresses systemic gaps by promoting

Key principle/pillar	Description
Owner-operator model	Nurse-owned and operated clinics serving underserved communities; nurses run clinics and handle primary care with referral pathways to doctors/hospitals; empowers nurses with clinic ownership, leading to quality service delivery.
Integrated care model	Patient-centric, holistic approach offering a wide range of primary care services (e.g., diagnosis, treatment, family planning, antenatal care, chronic illness, HIV counselling); reduces siloed care and wasteful expenditure.
Blended finance model	Mix of grant and loan funding; nurses repay loans over 5 years before gaining full ownership; includes impact equity, mezzanine debt, and loans; aims for financial sustainability while keeping care affordable.
Custom-designed software	Proprietary platform (WeCare) tailored for clinic operations: patient management, HR, finance, stock management, patient education, quality assessment, and virtual consultations; enhances clinic efficiency and data management.

Source: Adapted from Szerb et al. [22], Unjani Clinics NPC [34, 35], and Unjani Clinics [36].

Table 2.
Key principles and pillars of the Unjani Clinics model.

ownership and sustainability among nurses while enhancing service efficiency and patient outcomes. However, its long-term scalability depends on balancing financial viability with continued quality care delivery [22, 34, 36]. These clinics, supported through a blend of corporate social investment and nurse entrepreneurship, have successfully expanded to over one hundred operational sites nationally. Their decentralised structure enables flexible, localised health service delivery, demonstrating alignment with the WHO's HSS building blocks of service delivery and workforce development [36, 37]. Furthermore, they reflect key PHC values: community responsiveness, empowerment, and equity. However, the literature cautioned that sustainability depends on ongoing funding, mentorship, and regulatory support, especially in remote areas where health infrastructure is weakest [38, 39].

5.2 Improved access through retail health integration

Retail pharmacies such as Clicks and Dis-Chem have emerged as important non-traditional entry points into PHC [23, 24]. These outlets offer convenient walk-in services, including immunisations, screenings, and minor consultations, often during extended hours. Their integration with PHC aligns with the PHC principle of accessibility, particularly for employed individuals or those in peri-urban settings who may face barriers to accessing public clinics during standard working hours [40]. However, studies have also raised concerns about exclusionary effects due to affordability and medical scheme limitations, which risk reinforcing health inequities. These findings emphasise the need for policy oversight and inclusive pricing models to ensure retail health services contribute meaningfully to UHC goals [40].

5.3 Strategic resource optimisation via public-private partnerships

PPPs have emerged as a prominent strategy for optimising scarce healthcare resources, particularly in rural and under-resourced provinces with limited government capacity. Collaborations between government entities and private practitioners, such as general practitioners and obstetric and maternal care specialists, have proven instrumental in

Model	Key features	PHC and HSS alignment	Enablers	Challenges
Unjani Clinics	Nurse-led, integrated care, blended finance, custom tech (WeCare)	Equity, workforce, and community-based service	Social investment, mentorship	Funding gaps, rural infrastructure limits
Retail Clinics	Walk-in access, screenings, minor care, and use of commercial spaces	Accessibility, service convenience	Market demand, extended hours	Cost barriers, weak public system integration
PPPs	Contracted private providers, rural outreach, mixed financing	Workforce support, rural access, and UHC advancement	Governance frameworks, collaboration	Oversight gaps, policy misalignment

Table 3.
Conceptual model—private sector contributions to PHC and health systems strengthening in South Africa.

supplementing the public sector workforce. This augmentation has improved patient outcomes and reduced referral delays, addressing critical service delivery gaps [41].

Despite their growing recognition as essential tools for advancing UHC across Sub-Saharan Africa, PPPs face significant governance, regulatory oversight, and equitable access challenges. Otchere et al. [16] emphasise that, while PPPs hold immense potential for HSS, particularly in workforce development and service delivery pillars, their effectiveness is often hindered by weak policy alignment and insufficient capacity-building efforts. This critique points to systemic weaknesses that limit the scalability and sustainability of PPP initiatives.

Moreover, the variability in governance standards and contract terms, often marked by inadequate monitoring and evaluation frameworks, raises concerns about these partnerships' long-term impact and accountability. The literature suggests that PPPs risk perpetuating fragmentation within health systems without harmonised financing models, and more substantial alignment with national health policies [25, 41].

Further analysis by Ebulue, Ebulue, and Ekesiobi [42] reinforces that successful PPPs in global health innovation depend heavily on robust governance structures, genuine stakeholder collaboration, and clearly defined objectives. Their findings highlight transparency, contextual adaptation to local health environments, and sustained political and financial commitment as critical enablers for improving healthcare outcomes. This underscores the necessity for PPP frameworks that are not only well-designed but also dynamically responsive to evolving health system needs.

The conceptual framework emerging from this study, depicted in **Table 3** above, illustrates how private sector models, Unjani Clinics, retail health clinics, and PPPs contribute distinct, yet complementary, approaches to strengthening PHC and advancing UHC through service delivery, workforce development, and enhanced accessibility. While each model aligns with key PHC and HSS principles, their effectiveness and scalability are contingent upon enabling institutional factors, such as regulatory support, financing mechanisms, and governance structures, as well as their ability to overcome systemic challenges related to equity, integration, and sustainability.

6. Discussion

The findings from this literature review underscore the critical role that private sector innovations can play in strengthening South Africa's PHC system, particularly in addressing persistent gaps in service delivery, workforce capacity, and equitable access. Examining models, such as Unjani Clinics, retail health services, and PPPs, reveals insights into how private sector contributions complement and challenge the public health system's efforts to achieve UHC.

The success of the Unjani Clinics network in expanding access to primary care services in underserved communities exemplifies a scalable and sustainable model aligned with key PHC and HSS principles. As the literature suggests [22, 34, 36], empowering nurses through ownership and entrepreneurship fosters professional autonomy and service quality, addressing critical workforce shortages documented in the public sector [4, 5]. This aligns with the WHO's call for decentralised, community-based care that is person-centred and equitable [11]. The blend of social investment and innovative financing in the Unjani model reflects institutional pressures for financial viability balanced with social mission [43].

However, critical analysis indicates that sustainability is contingent on robust regulatory frameworks and continuous support, particularly in rural areas where infrastructure and supervision remain weak [38, 39]. This finding supports broader calls in the literature for deliberate policy alignment and stewardship to avoid fragmentation [15, 17]. It is evident that while nurse-led models advance PHC values, their integration within national health systems must be reinforced by governance mechanisms that safeguard quality and equity.

Retail pharmacy clinics represent an important innovation in enhancing PHC accessibility, particularly for working populations facing temporal and geographic barriers to public clinics [23, 24]. These models leverage existing commercial infrastructure to deliver a range of basic services, embodying the PHC tenet of accessibility and responsiveness [7]. Yet, the literature and this review highlight tensions between commercial motives and equitable service provision [20, 21]. Concerns about affordability and geographic distribution indicate retail clinics may inadvertently exacerbate inequities, reinforcing the dual health system dynamic where wealthier urban populations receive superior care.

This reflects institutional theory's insight that private actors must navigate competing normative demands between market efficiency and social accountability [43]. Thus, policy frameworks must ensure that retail health integration supports rather than undermines equity goals, through targeted subsidies or incentives for service provision in marginalised areas [44].

The review confirms that PPPs aim to alleviate human resource shortages and enhance quality, particularly in rural and underserved regions [25, 26]. Deploying private practitioners to support public facilities aligns with strengthening strategies for the health workforce within the WHO's HSS framework. However, the effectiveness of PPPs depends heavily on strong government stewardship, regulatory capacity, and alignment with national health priorities [15]. Findings reveal that PPPs risk perpetuating system fragmentation if not governed by transparent, accountable frameworks that promote shared objectives, rather than divergent sectoral interests [19]. This echoes prior literature emphasising the need for genuine trust-building, clear accountability, and community engagement to transcend mere transactional collaborations [20]. It highlights the institutional challenge of balancing legitimacy and compliance with innovation and sustainability goals. The alignment of private sector innovations with the WHO's HSS building blocks provides a useful heuristic for evaluating their systemic contributions and limitations. Service delivery and workforce development benefit from models like Unjani Clinics, yet information systems, governance, and financing elements require stronger integration and oversight.

This systemic perspective echoes the literature advocating for a systems-thinking approach, incorporating public and private actors as complementary, rather than competing, forces [15, 18].

Institutional theory further illuminates how regulatory, normative, and cognitive pressures influence the extent to which private innovations contribute to public health goals. For example, the Unjani model's embeddedness in a hybrid financing structure reflects a response to institutional demands for financial sustainability and social legitimacy [32, 34–36, 45]. Meanwhile, retail clinics' commercial orientation must be reconciled with health equity mandates through stronger normative and regulatory controls.

7. Limitations

While this review highlights promising private sector contributions, it also surfaces enduring equity, sustainability, and system coherence challenges. The dualistic nature of South Africa's health system, with a well-resourced private sector serving a minority, complicates integration efforts. The risk of exacerbating inequalities through market-driven models necessitates careful policy calibration to ensure that private sector innovations advance social justice and universal coverage goals. Moreover, the ongoing policy shift towards NHI presents an important context for future research. Understanding how private sector models can align with and complement NHI objectives is critical, particularly as new regulatory and financing mechanisms are introduced.

8. Recommendations

Several recommendations offer valuable lessons for other countries based on the study's key findings. First, to improve the scalability and sustainability of private sector initiatives such as Unjani Clinics, it is crucial to bolster public sector support through targeted funding, robust policy frameworks, and comprehensive capacity-building programmes. Encouraging greater collaboration between government and private nurse-led clinics can foster community ownership and ensure these models remain responsive to local health needs. Policymakers should also explore mechanisms to integrate such models formally into the national PHC framework to enhance coordination and resource allocation.

Regulatory frameworks should be updated to better accommodate the growing role of retail pharmacies in delivering primary health care services. This includes establishing clear quality and service delivery standards to protect patients and ensure continuity of care. Furthermore, equitable financing mechanisms, such as expanding insurance coverage or subsidising services, are needed to prevent these private retail-based services from deepening health disparities, ensuring they contribute effectively to universal health coverage goals.

Through strengthened governance structures and transparent contract management, PPPs must be supported to maximise their potential in addressing health workforce shortages and service gaps, especially in rural areas. Clear guidelines and monitoring systems should be developed to ensure PPPs align with national health priorities and maintain high-quality standards. Building trust and communication channels between public and private actors will be vital for long-term sustainability and system integration.

9. Conclusion

This study underscores the importance of partnerships and collaboration between the public and private sectors in advancing common public health goals, highlighting how innovative models such as nurse-led Unjani Clinics, retail pharmacy services, and public-private partnerships contribute to strengthening South Africa's primary health care system. These approaches have demonstrated potential in improving accessibility, scalability, and resource optimisation, addressing the public health sector's key challenges. To maximise their impact, future efforts should explore how such models can be effectively integrated into the broader health system to benefit the greater population and enhance equitable access to care. Their success will depend on appropriate policy alignment, regulatory oversight, and a shared commitment to equity and universal health coverage principles.

Acknowledgements and use of AI

While preparing this chapter, the authors utilised Grammarly and QuillBot for language editing, polishing, and plagiarism detection. All outputs generated by these tools were critically reviewed and edited by the author, who takes full responsibility for the final content presented in this publication.

Funding

No external funding was received to conduct this research or prepare the chapter.

Conflict of interest

The authors declare no conflicts of interest related to this study.

Data availability

The data used in this study were derived from secondary sources compiled through a comprehensive literature review. All data are publicly available and have been appropriately cited in the chapter.

Author details

Michael Mncedisi Willie*, Samantha Iyaloo, Kgothatso Nkoana, Phakamile Nkomo, Selby Masekela, Percy Daames and Musa Gumede
Council for Medical Schemes, Pretoria, South Africa

*Address all correspondence to: m.willie@medicalschemes.co.za

References

[1] Ataguba JE, McIntyre D. Paying for and receiving benefits from health services in South Africa: Is the health system equitable? Health Policy and Planning. 2012;**27**(Suppl 1):i35-i45. DOI: 10.1093/heapol/czs005

[2] Council for Medical Schemes (CMS). Industry Report 2024. Pretoria, South Africa: Council for Medical Schemes; 2024. Available from: https://www.medicalschemes.co.za/the-cms-2023-industry-report-is-here/

[3] Moeti T, King J, Padarath A, Ndlovu N, Mudau M, Chetty N. Profiling the unique passage of South Africa's health system reforms towards realisation of universal health coverage. The BRICS Health Journal. 2024;**1**(1):71-86. DOI: 10.47093/3034-4700.2024.1.1.71-86

[4] Maphumulo WT, Bhengu BR. Challenges of quality improvement in the healthcare of South Africa post-apartheid: A critical review. Curationis. 2019;**42**(1):1901. DOI: 10.4102/curationis.v42i1.1901

[5] van Weel C, Kidd MR. Why strengthening primary health care is essential to achieving universal health coverage. CMAJ. 16 Apr 2018;**190**(15):E463-E466. DOI: 10.1503/cmaj.170784. Available from: https://www.ncbi.nlm.nih.gov/pmc/articles/PMC5903888/

[6] Rai A, Khatri RB, Assefa Y. Primary health care systems and their contribution to universal health coverage and improved health status in seven countries: An explanatory mixed-methods review. International Journal of Environmental Research and Public Health. 2024;**21**(12):1601. DOI: 10.3390/ijerph21121601

[7] World Health Organization, United Nations Children's Fund (UNICEF). A Vision for Primary Health Care in the 21st Century: Towards Universal Health Coverage and the Sustainable Development Goals (WHO/HIS/SDS/2018.X). Geneva, Switzerland: World Health Organization; 2018. Available from: https://creativecommons.org/licenses/by-nc-sa/3.0/igo

[8] Alegre JC, Sharma S, Cleghorn F, Avila C. Strengthening primary health care in low- and middle-income countries: Furthering structural changes in the post-pandemic era. Frontiers in Public Health. 2024;**11**:1270510. DOI: 10.3389/fpubh.2023.1270510

[9] World Health Organization. Primary Health Care. Geneva, Switzerland: World Health Organization; 2025. Available from: https://www.who.int/news-room/fact-sheets/detail/primary-health-care

[10] Mofolo N, Heunis C, Kigozi GN. Towards national health insurance: Alignment of strategic human resources in South Africa. African Journal of Primary Health Care & Family Medicine. 2019;**11**(1):1928. DOI: 10.4102/phcfm.v11i1.1928

[11] Starfield B, Shi L, Macinko J. Contribution of primary care to health systems and health. Milbank Quarterly. 2005;**83**(3):457-502. DOI: 10.1111/j.1468-0009.2005.00409.x

[12] Behera BK, Prasad R, Shyambhavee. Primary health-care goal and principles. In: Healthcare Strategies and Planning for Social Inclusion and Development. Elsevier; 2021. pp. 221-239. DOI: 10.1016/B978-0-323-90446-9.00008-3

[13] Dookie S, Singh S. Primary health services at district level in

South Africa: A critique of the primary health care approach. BMC Family Practice. 2012;**13**(1):67. DOI: 10.1186/1471-2296-13-67

[14] Omoleke II, Taleat B. Contemporary issues and challenges of health sector in Nigeria. Research Journal of Health Sciences. 2018;5(4):210. DOI: 10.4314/rejhs.v5i4.5

[15] Naidoo V, Suleman F, Bangalee V. Medical insurance representatives perceptions on national health insurance primary healthcare re-engineering in South Africa: A qualitative study. Journal of Primary Care & Community Health. 2024;**15**:21501319241237044. DOI: 10.1177/21501319241237044

[16] Otchere G, Fusheini A, Sullivan T, Gauld R, Penno E. Public–private partnerships for universal health coverage in sub-Saharan Africa: A scoping review protocol. Health Science Reports. 2025;**8**(4):e70746. DOI: 10.1002/hsr2.70746

[17] Phua KH. Universal health coverage and public-private participation: Towards a new balance? Global Health Journal. 2017;**1**(2):3-11. DOI: 10.1016/S2414-6447(19)30078-8

[18] Bitton A, Ratcliffe HL, Veillard JH, Kress DH, Barkley S, Kimball M, et al. Primary health care as a foundation for strengthening health systems in low- and middle-income countries. Journal of General Internal Medicine. 2017;**32**(5):566-571. DOI: 10.1007/s11606-016-3898-5

[19] Brinkerhoff D. Accountability and health systems: Overview, framework, and strategies. In: The Partners for Health Reformplus Project. Cambridge, MA, USA: Abt Associates Inc.; 2003. Available from: https://www.globalhealthlearning.org/sites/default/files/reference-files/2.6Brinkerhoff_AccountabilityHealthSystemsOverview.pdf

[20] Bond W. Creating incentives for accountability in patient care. Virtual Mentor. 2013;**15**(6):522-528. DOI: 10.1001/virtualmentor.2013.15.6.pfor1-1306

[21] Jarawan E, Boiangiu M, Zeng W. Strengthening provider accountability: A scoping review of accountability/monitoring frameworks for quality of RMNCH care. PLOS Global Public Health. 2023;**3**(11):e0001968. DOI: 10.1371/journal.pgph.0001968

[22] Szerb A, Kivleniece I, Aggarwal V. Unjani clinics: Meeting the need for scale through social franchising. Journal of Organization Design. 2021;**10**(3-4):93. DOI: 10.1007/s41469-021-00106-2

[23] The Competition Commission (CompCom). Retail Pharmacy's Increasing Role in Primary Healthcare [Competition News, Edition 71]. Pretoria, South Africa: The Competition Commission; 2021. Available from: https://www.compcom.co.za/wp-content/uploads/2021/09/Competition-News-edition-71-September-2021.pdf

[24] Naidoo M. Primary Healthcare Clinic Market (Working Paper CC2023(01)). Pretoria, South Africa: Competition Commission of South Africa; 2023. Available from: https://www.compcom.co.za/wp-content/uploads/2023/09/Working-Paper_PHC_Clinic_20230903.pdf

[25] Kula N, Fryatt RJ. Public-private interactions on health in South Africa: Opportunities for scaling up. Health Policy and Planning. 2013;**29**(5):560-569. DOI: 10.1093/heapol/czt042

[26] Jensen J. A review of public–private partnership activities in health system strengthening. In: The Role of Public-Private Partnerships in Health Systems Strengthening: Workshop Summary

(Appendix a). Forum on Public-Private Partnerships for Global Health and Safety, Board on Global Health, Institute of Medicine, National Academies of Sciences, Engineering, and Medicine. US: National Academies Press; 2016. Available from: https://www.ncbi.nlm.nih.gov/books/NBK373286/

[27] World Health Organization. Monitoring the Building Blocks of Health Systems: A Handbook of Indicators and their Measurement Strategies. Geneva, Switzerland: WHO; 2010

[28] Witter S, Palmer N, Balabanova D, Mounier-Jack S, Martineau T, Klicpera A, et al. Health system strengthening—Reflections on its meaning, assessment, and our state of knowledge. The International Journal of Health Planning and Management. 2019;**34**(4):e1980-e1989. DOI: 10.1002/hpm.2882

[29] Manyazewal T. Using the World Health Organization health system building blocks through survey of healthcare professionals to determine the performance of public healthcare facilities. Archives of Public Health. 2017;**75**(1):50. DOI: 10.1186/s13690-017-0221-9

[30] World Health Organization. Declaration of Alma-Ata. In: International Conference on Primary Health Care, Alma-Ata, USSR, 6-12 September 1978. Geneva, Switzerland: World Health Organization; 1978 https://www.who.int/publications/almaata_declaration_en.pdf

[31] World Health Organization. Declaration of Astana: Global Conference on Primary Health Care, Astana, Kazakhstan, 25-26 October 2018 (WHO/HIS/SDS/2018.61). Geneva: World Health Organization; 2018. Available from: https://www.who.int/publications/i/item/WHO-HIS-SDS-2018.61

[32] Kraef C, Kallestrup P. After the Astana declaration: Is comprehensive primary health care set for success this time? BMJ Global Health. 2019;**4**(6):e001871. DOI: 10.1136/bmjgh-2019-001871

[33] Snyder H. Literature review as a research methodology: An overview and guidelines. Journal of Business Research. 2019;**104**:333-339. DOI: 10.1016/j.jbusres.2019.07.039

[34] Booth A, Sutton A, Papaioannou D. Systematic Approaches to a Successful Literature Review. 2nd ed. Thousand Oaks, CA: SAGE Publications; 2016

[35] Unjani Clinics NPC. About Unjani Clinics. n.d. Available from: https://unjani.org.za/about

[36] McGrath B. Professional nurse-led Unjani clinics: Empowering the nurse entrepreneur. Inquiry Journal (Durham (NH): Hamel Center for Undergraduate Research, University of New Hampshire). 6 Apr 2020;**2020**(6). Available from: https://scholars.unh.edu/inquiry_2020/6

[37] Raghavan R. Unjani clinic network: An innovative and scalable hybrid enterprise model that achieves social impact through entrepreneurship. Journal of Organization Design. 2021;**10**:11. DOI: 10.1007/s41469-021-00108-0

[38] Sarbasheva M, Makhieva Z, Maltsagova A, Khadzhieva L, Dzhafarov M. Sustainable development of primary health care systems. Reliability: Theory & Applications (RT&A). Dec 2024;**19**(Special Issue №6, Part-3):1602

[39] Muho A, Brugger C, Salzmann T, Wyss K, Steinmann P. Sustainability of health system strengthening interventions implemented at primary

healthcare level: A scoping review. BMJ Open. 2025;**15**(4):e095516. DOI: 10.1136/bmjopen-2024-095516

[40] Kenny K. The changing landscape of pharmacy accessibility. Pharmacy Times. 22 Jul 2025;**91**(7). Available from: https://www.pharmacytimes.com/view/the-changing-landscape-of-pharmacy-accessibility

[41] Tabrizi JS, Gharaee H. Public-private partnership policy in primary health care: A scoping review. Journal of Primary Care & Community Health. 2020;**11**:2150132720943769. DOI: 10.1177/2150132720943769

[42] Ebulue CC, Ebulue OR, Ekesiobi C. Public-private partnerships in health sector innovation: Lessons from around the world. International Medical Science Research Journal. 2024;**4**(4):484-499. DOI: 10.51594/imsrj.v4i4.1051

[43] Scott WR. Institutions and Organisations: Ideas, Interests, and Identities. 4th ed. Sage Publishing; 2014

[44] Wirtz V, Kaplan W, Cellini C. Use of retail pharmacies as a source of essential medicines, including family planning products, for public sector clients in low- and middle-income countries: a thought leadership paper. Arlington, VA: Management Sciences for Health; 2022. Prepared for the US Agency for International Development by the USAID Medicines, Technologies, and Pharmaceutical Services (MTaPS) Program. Available from: https://www.ghsupplychain.org/sites/default/files/2022-07/Use-of-retail-pharmacies-for-public-procurement-in-LMICs.pdf

[45] Sutherland M, Krige K. Unjani "clinics in a container": Social franchising in South Africa. Emerald Emerging Markets Case Studies. 2017;7(1):1-23. DOI: 10.1108/EEMCS-06-2016-0151

Section 2

Prevention and Non-communicable Disease Care across Populations

Chapter 3

Non-communicable Disease Prevention and Care in Community Oriented Primary Care (COPC): Lessons from South Africa

Peter Delobelle, Tumelo Assegaai, Ishaaq Datay, Darcelle Schouw, Naomi Levitt and Steve Reid

Abstract

Non-communicable diseases (NCDs) pose a significant and increasing burden to primary health services in low- and middle-income countries. Community-oriented primary care (COPC) offers an innovative way to tackling this challenge. The aim of this study was to identify and develop a feasible, acceptable and effective package of community-based NCD prevention and care activities embedded in COPC roll-out in socio-economically disadvantaged areas in Cape Town. The project was guided by community-based participatory research around two community health centres, one of which was a COPC learning site. Cooperative inquiry groups were established to co-design selected interventions and community health workers directed to run wellness hubs and manage diabetes and hypertension outside the health facilities. Processes were analyzed in terms of reach, effectiveness, adoption, implementation, and maintenance (RE-AIM), pointing to salient differences between the project sites. The COPC learning site showed potential for sustainability due to a higher perceived sense of local ownership, while in the other site, lack of role clarity, communication, accountability and a team approach all highlighted gaps in leadership capacity. These results highlight the importance of leadership and team building, community involvement and partnerships in developing community-based approaches towards sustainable NCDs prevention and care, indicating that COPC may constitute a suitable approach for reaching this objective.

Keywords: non-communicable diseases, prevention, care, community-oriented primary care, community-based participatory research, South Africa

1. Introduction

1.1 Burden of non-communicable diseases in South Africa

Non-communicable diseases (NCDs) pose a growing burden to health systems in low- and middle-income countries (LMICs), including South Africa [1], where NCDs have become the leading cause of mortality and account for almost 40% of deaths [2]. Strategies to shift the focus from largely curatively oriented health services towards community-based approaches for NCDs prevention and control are urgently needed, including task shifting of health services towards community health workers (CHWs) [3]. Current trends in health promotion emphasize community-based programmes, employing multiple activities spread over time, as well as community-based participatory research (CBPR) to ensure equal stakeholder partnerships across intervention levels [4].

Implementation research to strengthen health systems for NCDs is also needed [5]. By focusing on the delivery of effective interventions, implementation research driven by local priorities can improve the efficiency of resource allocation through identifying cost-effective and sustainable implementation strategies while achieving real-world impact. Implementation science can also be made participatory through prioritizing iterative and inclusive co-construction of knowledge and action between researchers and communities to advance equity and move towards decolonisation of global health [6].

1.2 Community orientated primary care as a strategic framework

Strengthening the quality, efficiency and equity of Primary Health Care (PHC) is a national priority in South Africa and several strategies have been suggested to revitalize PHC [7], including community-oriented primary care (COPC). COPC transforms the orientation of the health system from reactive facility-based primary care services that emphasize treatment of disease, to proactive community-based services that engage the whole population with an emphasis on health promotion and disease prevention [8]. COPC was pioneered in South Africa in the 1940s, but its concept abandoned during the apartheid era. It was later implemented in different countries worldwide, with successful outcomes in Brazil, but a systematic review conducted on its effectiveness showed that the concept is not fully implemented as envisaged and there is a need to evaluate its scale-up and effectiveness [9].

In the Cape Metro, Western Cape, South Africa, COPC was introduced in four learning sites in 2017 as part of the Ward-Based Outreach Teams approach, one of the pillars of National Health Insurance roll-out. The programme embraces five principles of comprehensive care, health equity, local resource analysis, practicing with science, and integrating services around the needs of users [10]. A programmatic process evaluation showed that implementation strategies varied across sites, with progress noted in terms of delineating scopes of practice, especially for CHWs, establishing relationships between facility- and community-based team members, but with clear gaps in defining roles and training needs [8]. More work is needed to enable community participation and stakeholder collaboration and more attention given to improved governance and change management in the functioning of appropriately trained and integrated PHC teams.

1.3 ACCELERATE study

The ACCELERATE study was funded by the Global Alliance for Chronic Diseases (GACD) through the South African Medical Research Council (SAMR) and conducted from Jan 2020 to July 2023 by the Chronic Diseases Initiative for Africa and Primary Health Care Directorate, University of Cape Town in partnership with researchers from the University of the Western Cape, Stellenbosch University and

University of Melbourne. The study aimed to leverage local and evidence-based interventions to strengthen community-based NCDs prevention and care embedded in the roll-out of COPC in the Cape Town Metro, supported by the Cape Town Metro Health Services.

The study applied CBPR in two PHC sites, of which one was a COPC learning site (BL). The COPC site had an estimated population of up to 54,006 according to the last official census [11] with a history rooted in apartheid, and characterized by lower socio-economic status and significant social challenges like gangsterism. The other site (RET) had an estimated population of 35,709 in the last census. Both sites consist of a predominantly mixed-race (Colored)[1] population (92%, resp. 87%) with Afrikaans being the main language. Both communities are located around 15 km from Cape Town.

The study design was informed by a framework for implementation and scale-up of population interventions for community settings (PRACTIS), integrated into a knowledge-to-action (KTA) cycle, which included integrated knowledge translation. Specific objectives included identifying community assets and enablers that would allow the programme to be rolled out, adapting the activities to the local context and conducting programme evaluation to assess barriers and facilitators for the scaling of activities.

The study was conducted in three phases (formative-intervention-evaluation), of which the first was significantly impacted by the Covid-19 pandemic and the need to rapidly appraise the effect of the pandemic on the management and control of NCDs at PHC level. Mixed methods results from this phase indicated that COPC offered a potentially innovative way to support integration of care and referral pathways between community- and facility-based services, with marked differences between the COPC learning site and the other site [12].

In the second phase, initiated at the end of Covid-19 restrictions, a cooperative inquiry group (CIG) was established in both study sites to plan the implementation of activities, in line with the original protocol. Each CIG consisted of facility-based health care workers, including the family physician, facility manager, nurses, CHWs and health committee members. They jointly developed a vision and mission and selected two interventions for action, community-based Wellness Hubs for NCDs prevention and care and a Care for the Carer programme. Activities included the development of referral criteria for patients to Wellness Hubs and self-management support guided by Western Cape on Wellness (WoW!), a transversal, wellness-promoting programme [13]. WoW! is driven by local champions and in this study included wellness interventions in each site supported by clinic health committees and WoW! stakeholders.

In the third and final study phases, phase two activities were evaluated using an evaluation framework from implementation science, and a facility survey was conducted on staff wellbeing, indicating priority areas for action. Objectives of this study were as follows:

- To describe the implementation of the ACCELERATE project in view of COPC rollout.
- To assess the appropriateness and acceptability of the selected intervention.

[1] Colored in South Africa refers to an ethnic group of mixed-race origin and specific cultural identity.

- To assess the factors that facilitated and/or hindered the process of implementation.
- To assess the reach and fidelity of implementing the selected interventions.
- To explore the sustainability of the selected interventions in both study sites.
- To summarize the lessons learnt and make recommendations for scale-up in the framework of COPC.

2. Method

2.1 Study design and framework

The study used a mixed methods design including quantitative data for Wellness Hub roll-out and attendance rates, and qualitative data to assess the participant perceptions. The latter were collected using a descriptive phenomenological approach [14], involving semi-structured interviews with key informants, focus group discussions with CIGs and patients living with NCDs, participant observation, and document analysis (meeting records, CIG diaries). The analysis was guided by the RE-AIM domains for programme evaluation (Reach, Effectiveness, Adoption, Implementation and Maintenance) [15], complemented by user perceptions of programme appropriateness and acceptability (**Table 1**).

Key informants included the Metro Health Services Chief Director, NCD Working Group Chair and Organizer, facility-based managers and staff, CHW managers and their staff, and family physicians (n = 13). Four focus group discussions were conducted with patients recruited from Wellness Hubs and CIG participants in both sites (n = 20). A purposive sample was used to recruit facility staff and CHWs, and

Domain	Description	Data source
Appropriateness/ acceptability	Acceptability of the programme and selected interventions	Key informant interviews Focus group discussions (patients)
Reach	Number of individuals who participated in the programme / intervention and perceived success	Wellness Hubs referral / attendance sheets Key informant interviews
Effectiveness	Perceived effectiveness of the programme and its interventions, including barriers and enablers	Key informant interviews Focus group discussions (CIGs)
Adoption	Perceived adoption of programme interventions and barriers / enablers	Key informant interviews
Implementation	Perceived success of programme roll-out and barriers / enablers of implementation of the selected interventions	Document analysis (meeting minutes, project documents) Participant observation (CIGs) Key informant interviews Focus group discussions (CIGs)
Maintenance	Perceived sustainability of the interventions and barriers / enablers	Key informant interviews Focus group discussions (CIGs)

Table 1.
RE-AIM domains operationalization and their respective data sources.

a convenience sample for patients and CIG participants. Eligibility criteria included participation in the ACCELERATE project, comprising facility managers, family physicians and CHWs who worked as part of COPC outreach teams, and patients with NCDs who attended the Wellness Hubs. Exclusion criteria included impaired decision-making capacity and need of urgent medical care. Patient sampling was considered to represent the range of NCDs patients in regard to age, gender, race, duration of living with NCDs, and receiving care.

2.2 Data collection

Data collection was informed by a (semi-) structured interview and focus group topic guide based on the indicators required for the RE-AIM framework evaluation. The guides were developed in English and translated into Afrikaans. A semi-structured format was used to capture a broad range of experiences and attitudes related to the study topic, while allowing participants to share their perspectives naturally and freely [16]. The topic guide was pilot tested with two health care workers, two CHWs, and two patients, to test the flow of questions, the relevance of probes, and the feasibility and acceptability regarding time and length of the interview. Findings from the pilot were used to refine and adapt the guides as necessary.

2.3 Data analysis

Data were analyzed using the thematic framework approach described by Pope & Mays [17] and thematic content analysis, guided by the RE-AIM framework for programme evaluation. A mixed deductive and inductive approach was used to identify pre-defined as well as emerging themes and categories. Interview and focus group recordings were professionally transcribed and checked for errors against the audio-recordings. Researchers familiarized themselves with the transcripts which were coded by two investigators, resulting in a list that was discussed with team members and compared for discrepancies until consensus was reached. Although codes were derived inductively from the data, the organization of codes was deductive to evaluate the different domains of the RE-AIM framework. All team members agreed on the final coding index, which was applied to the full set of transcripts for data extraction until saturation was reached. The analysis was triangulated through analysis of external meeting recordings and participant observations and supported by software for qualitative data analysis (NVivo9).

2.4 Ethics approval

Ethics approval was obtained from the Human Research Ethics Committee of the University of Cape Town (Ref 307/2020) and permission to conduct the study in the two facilities granted by the Western Cape Government Department of Health (Ref WC_202008_075). Confidentiality of study participants was maintained throughout data collection and analysis.

3. Results

Phase three results revealed variations in project implementation and goal achievement across sites. These differences underscored the importance of leadership, team building, community involvement and partnership, which shaped perceptions of local ownership and sustainability. Aspects of programme success (barriers and enablers) showed the impact of organizational culture, role clarity, teamwork, communication and accountability; the role of external facilitation as catalyst for teamwork and sustained programme planning (incl. Positionality of the researcher); the choice of selected interventions in line with local priorities (policy directions); the timing of activities in the immediate post-Covid era; and the effect of desirability bias in response to interviewer's questions in the evaluation phase.

3.1 Programme implementation

As regards implementation of the ACCELERATE programme, analysis of the semi-structured interviews with key informants and CIG participants based on the RE-AIM framework for programme evaluation revealed the following results.

As regards *implementation* form, the ACCELERATE programme was generally supported by respondents in terms of its *appropriateness and acceptability*, as illustrated by the following quote: *'I think because..., number one, we see the vision that you are coming with' (BL OPS)* and *'I also really appreciated the caring for the carer event that we had' (CIG Retreat).* Some reservations were made at the onset: *'I think by the time I arrived at the first meeting; I was not very happy. I thought that some people were stalling the process' (RET CBS Coord)* but the new way of working between facility and community was appreciated, as shown by the following quote: *'There was a lot of ideas that went around,... it was nice to get different viewpoints, from facility based staff and from community based staff' (RET CIG)* and *'I think we always engage with them as part of COPC but I think it just strengthens that relationship.' (BL SFP).*

As for its *effectiveness*, the programme seemed to have an impact on some respondents, as shown by the following quote: *'I think you opened my eyes, when you started ..., my eyes opened to really primary care of healthcare, ..you know, how we can actually make a difference' (RET HC)* and *'I think it brought a great understanding among each other because I would've gone freely to ... and tell her, listen here, there is a crisis or there is a problem, and she'll reply then to me and say yes, it was sorted and it makes everybody feel somebody is listening to what I'm saying.' (BL CIG).*

In terms of *adoption*, the COPC site showed consistent engagement with the programme, as illustrated by: *'I think the running of the meetings went well, especially the fact that people could come and express how they feel, they could feel comfortable to say, and as I said, I liked the build-up of the project when you initially started, how you eased everybody into it to say this is what the project is all about, we want to make a difference, what is your goal, what is your vision and how do we want to achieve it. (BL, MGR)*, while the non-COPC site featured less support: *'Not so much support from the facility... we've had them once or twice, I think' (RET OTL).*

In terms of programme *sustainability*, there were marked differences between both sites, as shown by these quotes: *'I think that, from these meetings, that is something that is carried forward. It's..., just the fact that it started here, it went out to the community, and we got the community starting to get involved,' (RET CIG)* and *'Seeing that these ladies are working in the community, that we probably would be the champion amongst them so they can also ... sort of drive this' (BL CIG).* Some of this may be attributed to factors related to the internal context, as shown for example by this quote: *'We had a meeting and that's something ...we picked up, in terms of the handover; the orientation. How would you expect me to deliver... good quality if you don't orientate and then you don't hand over,' (BL OPS)* and *'They do tick sheets and tick boxes very well, but they don't do leadership very well.' (RET FP).*

3.2 Programme interventions

For programme intervention, the sites prioritized risk stratification, decentralizing care to the community, and the Care for the Carer programme. These choices aligned with the Cape Town Metro Chronic Diseases Working Group objectives for reorganizing services and recruitment of WoW! Champions in each sub-District. The former was implemented as Wellness Hubs were rolled out in each sub-District and the latter linked to the implicit objective of staff and patient health and wellbeing. Both interventions are described in more detail in the next section.

3.2.1 Wellness hubs

Analysis of interview transcripts related to the Wellness Hubs intervention (**Table 2**) revealed that the programme faced a learning curve but was considered successful (*appropriateness/acceptability*), especially in the COPC (BL) site: *'I thought it was going to be more difficult than what I expected because, but okay, I'm not a clinician, but I thought, in my mind I thought, wow, this is going to be a shift from what we know and, and then as time went along, I saw almost a..., it can be done, it's doable.'*

Theme	Category	Quote
Appropriateness	Convenience	'I would say this is a great success because it is closer to patient's houses. They do not, and some of them have to take a taxi to the facility, so now they just walk to the club.' (BL CPN)
	Acceptability	'Wider range and they actually love the way we are doing the BMIs and stuff now. And then... the health education is going on and I think it's much better because the facility ... the atmosphere or what can a person say, the environment at the facility is too clinical.' (RET OTL)
	Facility decongestion	'It's a good thing. It's going to help the clinic as well with this thing. Then you can focus more on patients who really do need your care or that you need to refer.' (BL CPN)
Reach	Safety	'Patients are really complaining, because they say it's territory related. Half of them come halfway ... and they get chased back because people think they are coming to spy there, the gangsters and then there is a fight about anything.' (BL CPN)
	Logistical concerns	'Sometimes I do not know if it's the taxi fare, or it's too far for them to walk, so they have their own reasons. I do not think the community health workers actually went so far and asked them why are they not coming?' (RET OTL)
Effectiveness	Collaboration	'it's like there's a an organization that can help you. ... I do not have to go waste the social worker's time now, she's busy enough trying to find her intermediate care facility for a patient with bed sores, kind of scenario..' (RET FP)
	Integration / communication	'So, yeah, it was a good team vibe in this space. We didn't have any like really,... we didn't have a lot of fighting, arguing... people will try to understand this one's circumstance and why it was difficult and find solutions to the problems.' (BL CIG)
	Barriers	'I think there are lots of ... I guess what I'm trying to say is there are lots of factors that make us inefficient. We do not have enough connections with what's out there in the community and to the resources that's available to us.' (RET FP)

Theme	Category	Quote
Adoption	Role of manager	'I think for me... as a manager, ... unfortunately you must have your finger in all the pies because if you do not, things fall flat, so for me, I saw this golden opportunity of a partner, a stakeholder, supporting me to make sure that someone is going forward.' (BL MGR)
	Conceptualization	'I think for me it was a good experience because what we ultimately would like to achieve or partially achieved with ACCELERATE and the support of the team was to get the service closer to the patient.' (BL MGR)
	Shared vision	'The fact that people are busy making plans to improve the health of the community, that is something that is very welcoming and what, there was actually nothing that I didn't experience as not acceptable because I know it's a work in progress.' (BL HLTH PROM)
	Stakeholder engagement	'It was just Sister X basically..., the councilor just helped with venues, basically, and as you say, the volunteers have now come on to help with the patient flow.' (BL MGR)
	Facilitation	'I saw this opportunity to capitalize on the knowledge, what you guys were bringing to the table and the support that we were getting to be able to make the hubs a success, I do not think we would have been able to do it so quickly.' (BL MGR)
Implementation	Teamwork	'There was a lot of work put in by a lot of people... to get these hubs going and I think that helps any project to see if you have someone who's, who's putting a lot of effort, a lot of time into it to also get it to work.' (BL CIG)
	Facilitation	'I really liked the way you came in and started talking about what the goals and objectives were, it was not something that was dumped on us and you have to run with it – it made the team think of, what do we actually want to achieve.' (BL MGR)
	Barriers	'The attendance was really erratic and I think that was the main challenge. .. I think there were teething problems in the beginning with the doctor sending patients over and they do not go over, they go home. That's what happened.' (RET OTL)
Maintenance	Policy	'...this is also part of the department's differentiated models of care systems, ... where you are not only providing services at the facility but you are also providing services outside, like the e-lockers, the medication drop-offs.' (BL MGR)
	Management	'It's definitely sustainable, because if you are not going to ensure that your staff is cared for the project is not going to work, if you are not going to listen to their concerns and make sure that their wellbeing is catered for, you are not going to succeed.' (BL MGR)
	Workload / resources	'I also feel that the facility must bring some sort of ... not responsibility, but sometimes it becomes a norm, it's your problem ... at the moment, it seems that everything is about hubs, but we ... as community health workers, we have much more than just hubs.' (RET CIG)
	Opportunities	'I just think the community awareness, maybe a little bit more of media involvement, ... Possibly get a bit more stakeholders on board, get the religious leaders... so that the broader community is aware of what is happening.' (BL MGR)

Table 2.
RE-AIM domains (themes), categories, and quotes for programme intervention.

(BL CIG FGD). The intervention was seen as convenient to patients and decongesting facilities: *'They really appreciate the hub now, because it's one step in and one step out.' (BL, CBS).* In the non-COPC site, feelings were more mixed: *'Yeah, I guess it's like, is it realistic to expect patients who are living in that dire circumstance, to worry about what is going to be like in two years' time?'* and *'Is it realistic to expect the healthcare worker, who is in a meeting, dealing with emergencies constantly, and doing crisis management, to worry about the HbA1c control of diabetics?' (RET FP).*

Programme roll-out (*reach*) was slightly hampered by safety and logistical concerns due to the location and physical state of some community venues, and the pace of roll-out differed substantially between sites, with the COPC learning site reporting seven established hubs between March-July 2023 and the non-COPC learning site only one. Monthly attendance rates varied from 45 to 287 patients in the COPC site, versus 58–73 in the non-COPC site. The difference was likely due to variations in collaboration and teamwork in both sites, as shown in the paragraphs below, with the COPC site showing more cohesion and ability to coordinate programme roll-out than the non-COPC site. The COPC site was also more expressive and engaged in the intervention than the non-COPC site: *'Can I just add to that, and before it wasn't like that. It's like we were different entities, like we were careful of each other and so now suddenly there's a, like, we are closer and we don't mind to ask a question.' (BL CIG).*

The perceived *effectiveness* of the intervention was influenced by the end of Covid-related home delivery of medication, which interfered with the process as shown by the following quote: *'I think it was running smoother until they stopped the home deliveries and that threw a massive wrench in the implementation of our system... and so with that, and even now as you say, we're still getting a lot of people coming here instead of the hub, so we still have a lot of implementation struggles' (BL CIG).* This however changed over time, as shown by the following: *'But actually, if I look at the ... compared to the first like three or four months that the hubs were open to the next like two or three months that have gone by, a lot more people are open to it and accept that idea and are willing to go to the hubs.' (BL FP).*

Implementation of the hubs was facilitated by the CIG stakeholders, and activities varied from marketing the hubs in and outside the facility by health care workers and community health workers, securing sites by the local community leader, and willingness of the nurses to move services to these hubs. Developing a shared vision and engaging stakeholders proved to be crucial for the *adoption* of the intervention, facilitated by the research team and management support: *'Yes, I liked that build up to the whole thing, I liked that, the fact that people were taken into where are we going to with this' (BL MGR);* and *'Patients that didn't want to understand at first what the wellness hub is... so look we have to make them understand...' (BL MGR).*

Meanwhile, the non-COPC site faced issues of leadership and role clarity: *'I don't know if it is lack of human resources, for example I have this vision that at the wellness hub in the afternoon we could have immunizations, we could have woman's health and child health. But it seems to me that the facility doesn't grasp..., so understand that. So, we need to, I am sure because there is no staff to come out.' (RET CBS COORD).* There was also animosity among managers and CHWs in this site, as shown for example by the following: *'And then it's a ... ... I guess what I'm trying to say is there are lots of factors that make us inefficient. We don't have enough connections with what's going out there in the community and to the resources that's available to us' (RET FP)* and *'To me ... they did not really manage because they didn't do it as frequently as like me and the other CHWs that was this side, did it.' (RET CBS).*

The different pace of intervention roll-out and perceived support, teamwork, and collaboration translated into differences in perceived sustainability between both sites (*maintenance*). The continuity of hubs was deemed possible over time because it was part of a systems strategy, although there were legal concerns related to labour regulations when working outside the facility premises: '*The union said I'm not covered. If anything should happen, I'm not covered... but then now I, no, I'm not covered if anything should happen to me.*' *(BL CPN)*. Safety and security concerns also arose as the sites often experienced violent gang-related activities. Other issues related to staff shortage in the facility, resulting in nurses being unable to assist with work taking place in the hubs.

Overall, however, the programme roll-out was perceived to be valuable and aligned with current policy: '*well most definitely on the hubs, there's no plan to essentially shut them down at any point soon and ...I think a meeting of this kind of nature is a necessity to sort of keep them going... we will most definitely be continuing the mission, meetings unless they decide to scrap the idea of the hubs itself cause that's sort of our main focus from the community oriented approach.*' *(BL CIG)*. The feeling among CIG respondents was also positive, in that: '*...the more we come together and the more concerns we raise, the quicker we can fix everything, because we can't wait until the next month and if we must still wait another month to fix that problem, it's too long.*' *(BL CIG)*.

3.2.2 Caring for the carer

The Caring for the Carer programme, which included physical activity sessions and health status measurements of facility and community workers, was well perceived and appreciated, as shown by the following: '*I also really appreciated the caring for the carer event that we had. I don't think, I speak under correction, that the NPO, the carers and the staff has come together to have something*' *(RET CIG)* and: '*It was a good programme. Care for the carer. Yes. Somebody that looks after us*' *(BL CPN)* and: '*It was really appreciated by a lot of staff, that got to have their measurements done and got to see ... and they got to like stalls and stands and knowledge about that.*' *(BL FP)*. In the non-COPC site, the process was derailed by internal dynamics: '*Let me go back to the care for the carer. At the end of the day, I want to say that's lacking because we've always had that partnership but now it's business, so I am meeting a new person and it is almost you making a nuisance because that person annoys me and now there is an interim person, and the question is why is there an interim person?*' *(RET CBS COORD)*. In the COPC site, roll-out of the programme was, however, also affected by a change in management: '*The new management that has taken over, there has been communication that, ... you need to wear your uniform, you can't exercise like in, you can't come to work in tracksuits, if you do, you need to change your clothes, you need to have the epaulettes on and stuff like that, also you need to go back to your work area afterwards. So that has actually deterred staff a little bit because I think there hasn't been enough managers attending and driving this process.*' *(BL FP)*.

4. Discussion

Results from this study indicate that there was a salient difference between the two study sites: one in which there was integrated leadership and teamwork, and which built on the experience of being a COPC learning site for at least 3 years. In the COPC site, facility managers worked closely with community-based services, a relationship that was strengthened rather than weakened by Covid-19 [12, 18]. This was contrasted by the non-COPC site, where lack of role clarity, communication and accountability, and lack of a team approach, characterized by blaming and finger-pointing, highlighted gaps in leadership capacity. As one of the interviewees put it, there are 'too many managers and not enough leaders here'. By contrast with the COPC learning site, there was no history of explicit attempts to implement a COPC approach, as it was not identified as a COPC learning site in the Cape Town Metro.

Community involvement in the process was patchy and inconsistent in the non-COPC site, indicating lack of full community ownership of the programme, except at some later established peripheral hubs where patients started taking responsibility for some activities alongside the NGO. This could be expected, because communities are diverse and heterogeneous, with different forces pulling in different directions. In the COPC site, there was also evidence of strong intersectoral support, for example from police services in ensuring safety at the wellness hubs. In terms of the concept, community ownership hence started to be realized in the site that was designated a COPC learning site, but less in the other. The Caring for the Carer intervention also succeeded or foundered, respectively, on the level of management support. Where managers saw its benefit and supported activities personally, it became sustainable.

As indicated by the programme evaluation of COPC implementation in the Cape Town Metro Health District [8], understanding COPC and its underlying philosophy contrasts with the traditional model of care. The model requires strong leadership, and community and stakeholder engagement to bring about the required paradigm shift. In their evaluation, Goliath et al. [8] noted that the aim of team integration was not achieved to the same degree across the four investigated COPC sites. Some NGOs reported a sense of separation of responsibilities which weakened relationships and hindered team integration. They highlighted the importance of trust and clearly defined roles and responsibilities, which was also found in our study and reinforces the notion of sustained stakeholder engagement with community-based service providers.

With respect to the effect of the project itself on interventions, both positive and negative aspects might be seen as limitations of this study. Covid-19 disruptions and the post-Covid phase meant there was less time for implementation than originally envisaged (18 months instead of 36 months). In addition, and in agreement with the Metro Chief Director, only two sites were identified for programme implementation rather than four, which limited the diversity of experiences. There were significant changes in facility management in both sites during the project period; hence, teams were not entirely stable. The limitations, however, played out differently in both sites, as the COPC site was more prepared to deal with these challenges through adaptive management and solid community partnerships.

Through their consistent presence, the research investigators who facilitated the CIGs also created a space where people could interact, allowing internal role-players to speak to each other in front of an audience, including community members, which had a positive effect on teamwork in both sites. Facilitators were aware of the effect of their position as interviewers on the data being collected, and the desirability bias that resulted in people saying what they thought interviewers wanted to hear which could be perceived as a study limitation.

The factors described above also affected programme sustainability, which seemed to be more feasible in the COPC site but not the non-COPC site, despite a change in management in both. Perceived management support, teamwork, and collaboration in the COPC site translated into more realistic perceptions of sustainability and the continuity of hubs a real possibility over time. Finally, and in terms of NCDs control, measurements of hypertension and diabetic control over time were not done due to the limited project duration but could be assessed in further research.

5. Relating findings to change theory

The changes witnessed in both sites can be further explained with change theory, including the theory of diffusion of innovations and social support theory.

5.1 Diffusion of innovations theory

The diffusion of innovations theory states that for any new idea to take root, time is required. The idea is usually initiated by innovators and initially taken up by early adopters, followed by an early and then late majority. Invariably, a group of people remains who will continue to resist the idea (laggards). Between the early adopters and early majority there can be a schism or a barrier to adoption. This barrier can be challenging to bridge due to a lack of evidence generation, reduction of cost or effort needed to assimilate the innovation [19]. Sometimes change can also be initiated as a result of crisis.

In this study, both facilities faced the challenge of the Covid-19 pandemic and the response to change was quite evident. The facility that was already exposed to the COPC model was able to quickly leverage the previously established networks into a comprehensive response, while the non-COPC site needed to craft solutions without prior learning. The COPC site hence included innovators and early adopters, and the crisis allowed a bridging of the gap to reach an early majority. The Social Support theory can help to explain this in more detail as the COPC site acted as an early adopter that helped facilitate change management.

5.2 Social support theory

Social Support theory states that to achieve change at network or organizational level, informational, appraisal, emotional as well as instrumental support is needed [20]. CHWs are a well-known source of social support and providers of NCDs care at PHC level [21]. Social support is multidimensional and linked to the concept of social capital, in which social support and social networks are key. Both can be structurally and functionally embedded, either formally or informally, and constitute a building block for the development of social capital [22]. The theory of social relationships developed by Weiss [23] also focuses on the individual need to interact with other persons.

COPC supports community involvement in PHC service delivery and contributes to building social networks, which was evident in this study by comparing outcomes in terms of shared NCDs management between facility and community-based health workers in the COPC vs. non-COPC learning site, regardless of the support offered by study investigators who facilitated social bonds in both sites by providing a platform for meeting and interaction. The research team played an active role in establishing and strengthening connections by organizing monthly meetings at times and venues that were convenient, offered in an off-site venue and supported by light catering to shape a relaxed atmosphere, all of which can be described as *instrumental* support.

In addition, information on COPC, stakeholder mapping, and wellness hubs was provided through stakeholder teams or as a result of CIG members interacting with each other during meetings, which can be seen as example of *informational* support. Members who attended the meeting were also able to share challenges and success stories they were experiencing and benefitted from the listening ears of those who were in attendance (*emotional* support). Feedback on progress was constantly given and would instil further action, which would be fed back at the next meeting. This is an example of *appraisal* support, all of which was facilitated by the implementation of CBPR in both sites, which seemed more hands-on in the COPC vs. non-COPC site.

Hence, and in summary, it could be argued that COPC actively contributed to the creation of social support which, in turn, facilitated the NCDs management at local level. This could translate into the recommendation to roll out COPC to other non-learning sites, in order for the shift from curative services to community-based prevention to materialize in other sites. Further research is, however, needed within the context of CBPR and implementation research, underpinned by theoretical bases found within health promotion and social behavioral theories of change to elaborate this point.

6. Conclusion

As this study indicated, the quality and depth of leadership and building trust for sustained community involvement within COPC helped to create an environment that is conducive for innovation and adaptation in a PHC setting. The original project plan aimed to establish more community engagement in health services delivery, anticipating some degree of adjustment, but when forcefully disrupted by Covid-19, an even greater level of adaptation to change was needed. Through the contrasting experiences in the two project sites, it became clear that COPC led to more reach and adoption of strategies involving communities, better implementation and perceived effectiveness, and more realistic prognosis of sustainability, which may act as a suitable conduit for community-wide improvements in NCDs control, despite the challenges and constraints facing the current health system and the time needed to fully develop these improvements.

Despite the specific characteristics of both study sites in terms of socio-economic and historical development, the findings show promise for wider application of, and scale-up of the model. They unequivocally point to the potential impact of COPC in achieving decentralized services delivery in terms of NCDs control, with wider repercussions in terms of resilience in the face of adversity and disruption of fragile health systems in the region. The implications of facilitating COPC roll-out can also help inform similar initiatives at wider scale to achieve health systems objectives in an efficient and timely manner, inspired by the pivotal work done around COPC in South Africa and elsewhere.

Acknowledgements

The authors wish to acknowledge the support and contribution of Western Cape Metro Health Services in the conceptualisation of this study; the assistance of facility managers in both study sites to organize data collection and the assistance of facility and community-based healthcare workers, their managers, and all the patients who participated in this study.

Funding

The ACCELERATE project 'Assessing COPC scale-up in selected learning sites of the Cape Town Metro: Community-based NCD prevention interventions' was funded by the Global Alliance for Chronic Diseases (GACD) through a grant received from the South African Medical Research Council (SAMRC) (Ref 3233/CO284/KS/2019).

Conflict of interest

The authors declare no conflict of interest.

Author details

Peter Delobelle[1,2]*, Tumelo Assegaai[1], Ishaaq Datay[1], Darcelle Schouw[3], Naomi Levitt[1] and Steve Reid[1]

1 University of Cape Town, Cape Town, South Africa

2 Vrije Universiteit Brussel, Brussels, Belgium

3 Stellenbosch University, Cape Town, South Africa

*Address all correspondence to: peter.delobelle@uct.ac.za

References

[1] Mayosi BM, Flisher AJ, Lalloo UG, Sitas F, Tollman SM, Bradshaw D. The burden of non-communicable diseases in South Africa. The Lancet. 2009;**374**(9693):934-947

[2] Stats SA. Non-communicable Diseases in South Africa: Findings from Death Notifications 2008-2018. Pretoria: Statistics South Africa; 2023

[3] Haregu T, Delobelle P, Shrestha A, Panniyammakal J, Thankappan KR, Parasuraman G, et al. The shifting roles of community health workers in the prevention and management of noncommunicable disease during COVID-19 pandemic: A scoping review. Health Policy and Planning. 2024;**39**(7):771-781

[4] Hassan S, Kagwanja N, Diallo B, Oyando R, Perel P, Etyang A, et al. Implementing community-based interventions for the management of chronic conditions in low- and middle-income countries: A scoping review of qualitative evidence. PLOS Global Public Health. 2025;**5**(7):e0004860

[5] Rasanathan K, Dako-Gyeke P, Isaranuwatchai W, Mahendradhata Y, Roberts M, Loffreda G, et al. Non-communicable diseases: Can implementation research change the game for policy and practice? Lancet. 2024;**404**(10466):1908-1910

[6] The Lancet Global Health. Redefining implementation science for global health decolonisation. The Lancet Global Health. 2025;**13**(4):e599

[7] Schneider H, Jabulani M, Morewane R, Perez G. Primary health care. In: Matsoso M, Chikte U, Makubalo L, Pillay Y, Fryatt R, editors. The South African Health Reforms 2015-2020: The Road Ahead. Cape Town: UCT; 2022. pp. 58-80

[8] Goliath C, Mash R, Mahomed H. The implementation of community-oriented primary care in the cape metro Health District: A programme evaluation. South African Medical Journal. 2025;**115**(2):e2557

[9] Mash B, Ray S, Essuman A, Burgueno E. Community-orientated primary care: A scoping review of different models, and their effectiveness and feasibility in sub-Saharan Africa. BMJ Global Health. 2019;**4**(Suppl 8):e001489

[10] Mash R, Goliath C, Mahomed H, Reid S, Hellenberg D, Perez G. A framework for implementation of community-orientated primary care in the metro health services, Cape Town, South Africa. African Journal of Primary Health Care & Family Medicine. 2020;**12**(1):e1-e5

[11] Statistics South Africa: Census 2011. Pretoria: Statistics South Africa; 2011

[12] Delobelle PA, Abbas M, Datay I, De Sa A, Levitt N, Schouw D, et al. Non-communicable disease care and management in two sites of the Cape Town metro during the first wave of COVID-19: A rapid appraisal. African Journal of Primary Health Care & Family Medicine. 2022;**14**(1):e1-e7

[13] Western Cape Department of Health: Western Cape on Wellness (WOW!): Creating a Culture of Wellness Together. Annual Report 2018. Western Cape Department of Health: Cape Town; 2019

[14] Beck CT. Phenomenology: Its use in nursing research. International Journal of Nursing Studies. 1994;**31**(6):499-510

[15] Glasgow RE, Harden SM, Gaglio B, Rabin B, Smith ML, Porter GC, et al. RE-AIM planning and evaluation framework: Adapting to new science and practice with a 20-year review. Frontiers in Public Health. 2019;7(64)

[16] Beebe J. Basic concepts and techniques of rapid appraisal. Human Organization. 1995;**54**(1):42-51

[17] Pope C, Ziebland S, Mays N. Qualitative research in health care: Analysing qualitative data. British Medical Journal. 2000;**320**(7227):114-116

[18] Mash RJ, Schouw D, Daviaud E, Besada D, Roman D. Evaluating the implementation of home delivery of medication by community health workers during the COVID-19 pandemic in Cape Town, South Africa: A convergent mixed methods study. BMC Health Services Research. 2022;**22**(1):98

[19] Rogers EM. Diffusion of Innovations. 5th ed. Riverside, United States: Free Press; 2003

[20] Drageset J. In: Haugan G, Eriksson M, editors. Social Support. In: Health Promotion in Health Care - Vital Theories and Research. Cham (CH): Springer; 2021. pp. 137-144

[21] Longhini J, Canzan F, Mezzalira E, Saiani L, Ambrosi E. Organisational models in primary health care to manage chronic conditions: A scoping review. Health & Social Care in the Community. 2022;**30**(3):e565-e588

[22] Putnam R. Making Democracy Work. Princeton, NJ: Princeton University Press; 1993

[23] Weiss RS. Continuities and transformations in social relationships from childhood to adulthood. In: Hartup WW, Rubin Z, editors. Relationships and Development. New York: Psychology Press; 1986. pp. 95-110

Chapter 4

Ward-Based Community Healthcare Workers' Challenges Regarding the Utilization of Non-communicable Diseases Screening Tools, Limpopo Province, South Africa

Irene Ramavhoya Thifhelimbilu and Melitah Rasweswe Molatelo

Abstract

Screening is vital in detecting potential problems early, and it allows for timely intervention or specialized services. The South African Department of Health, in alignment with the World Health Organization's initiative, has appointed community healthcare workers through the primary healthcare reengineering programme to screen patients in the community. The main goal of their appointment was to screen the members of households to reduce the burden caused by quadruple diseases such as diabetes mellitus and hypertension. Regardless, community healthcare workers are faced with multiple challenges. As such, the current study was conducted to explore and describe the challenges experienced by ward-based community healthcare workers when using patient screening tools. A qualitative exploratory descriptive research design was used. Data was collected through focus group discussions with ten participants in each group, who were sampled purposively. Thematic analysis was used to analyse data. Three themes with six sub-themes emerged from the data. The findings revealed challenges related to community healthcare workers, as limited scope of practice, poor recognition, inadequate cooperation, distrust among patients and family members, and a shortage of screening tools and equipment. In conclusion, the unavailability of resources, family distrust, and limited scope had a negative impact on the implementation of the primary reengineering program and hampered the identification of family members at risk of non-communicable diseases. As such, community awareness of community healthcare workers' activities in the ward was recommended to ensure their acceptance.

Keywords: ward-based, community healthcare workers, screening tools, challenges, non-communicable diseases

1. Introduction

In South Africa, ward-based community healthcare workers (WBCHWs) are tasked with the responsibility of utilizing the screening tools when visiting patients in their homes [1]. This followed the initiative made by the World Health Organization (WHO), which planned a package of essential non-communicable disease interventions for primary healthcare facilities [2]. This package is to be utilized by ward-based community health workers (WBCHWs) all over the globe [3]. As a result, engagement with the local community facilitators was initiated, and South Africa developed the primary healthcare reengineering framework and strategy. This resulted in the appointment and training of WBCHWs who serve to support the distribution of primary healthcare services within the context of National Health Insurance [3, 4]. The main aim of appointing them was to reduce the burden caused by quadruple diseases, such as non-communicable diseases, which include diabetic mellitus and hypertension, through screening [5]. Diabetic mellitus accounts for more than 40% of adults, with hypertension accounting for more than 50% of the condition and the most common cause of death globally, including South Africa [5–7]. Regardless, WBCHWs are faced with multiple challenges during the process of implementing screening tools. In Sub-Saharan countries, a shortage of health care providers, such as nurses, has led to WHCHWs providing service to a region that carries 24% of the global burden of disease, leading to a high workload on their side [7]. Furthermore, the challenges they experience were influenced by social conditions, mental health status of the patient, patient adherence to medication, communication, and work environment [7, 8]. A synthesis was conducted on the experiences of CHCWs in countries such as India, Bangladesh, Pakistan, Sierra Leone, Kenya, and Ethiopia, where access and attitudes of the community, distrust, and stigmatization had an impact on the utilization of the screening tool [8, 9].

In South Africa, analysis of data from other studies revealed that WBCHWs are often faced with socioeconomic challenges in their line of work, whereby WBCHWs travel a long distance and pay for transport to visit patients who reside far from the clinic [10]. This had a negative impact on their services, which include visiting households for screening purposes. In Limpopo, most of the WBCHWs are generally poor with a low level of payment that limits their ability to access basic sites, WBCHWs reported that sometimes they have to pay from their own pockets to help their patients for transport to go to a clinic, placing further strain on their minimal resources [11]. As a result, this study was conducted to explore and describe the challenges experienced by the WBCHWs regarding the utilization of non-communicable diseases screening tools at Limpopo Province, South Africa.

2. Materials and methods

2.1 Study design

A qualitative exploratory descriptive research design was used to explore and describe the challenges experienced by the WBCHWs regarding the utilization of non-communicable diseases screening tools at Limpopo Province, South Africa.

2.2 Study setting

The study was conducted in the Limpopo Province, one of the rural provinces in the northeast corner of South Africa. Limpopo Province has a population of 5.5

million people and 290,521 households [12]. Limpopo has five districts consisting of Capricorn, Vhembe, Mopani, Waterberg, and Sekhukhune with 22 sub-districts. The Sekhukhune district consists of Elias Motsoaledi, Ephraim Mogale, Makhuduthamaga, and the Fetakgomo-Tubatse sub-districts. This study was conducted in selected primary healthcare facilities of the Fetakgomo-Tubatse sub-district, which consists of seven PHC facilities namely: Burgersfort, Mecklenburg Gateway, Selala, H.C Boshoff Health Centre, Dilokong Gateway, Madiseng Satellite, and Riba. In this study, only three PHC facilities were selected. This location was chosen on the basis that it has consistently retained WBCHWs since 2012 and has the greatest number of households (125,361) in any other sub-district.

2.3 Population and sampling

All elements (people, objects, events, or substances) that satisfy the sample requirements for research inclusion are referred to as the population [13]. This study used all trained WBCHWs who are utilizing non-communicable screening tools from the Fetakgomo-Tubatse sub-district, Limpopo Province as the population. The study employed a non-probability criterion purposive sampling design, with participants intentionally selected for inclusion in the sample based on the researcher's understanding of the population [14, 15]. Therefore, in the study, forty (40) trained ward-based community health workers were sampled purposively as the researcher knew that they were utilizing non-communicable screening tools when visiting patients and households. Those who were willing to participate were included in the study.

2.4 Data collection and analysis

Data collection is the systematic gathering of data related to a study's aims, questions, or hypotheses [15]. The researcher used a focus group interview guide to collect data from the participants. The reason for using the FGDs was to generate details of the challenges experienced by WBCHWs regarding the utilization of non-communicable screening tools related to diabetic mellitus and hypertension. This was to identify patients who might be at risk and those suffering from non-communicable diseases (diabetes mellitus and hypertension) during the household visits.

2.5 Preparation for data collection

2.5.1 Recruitment of participants

After obtaining permission to conduct the study from the Limpopo provincial Department of Health, Sekhukhune district, and the PHC facilities where data were collected, the researcher started the process of recruiting participants. The researcher communicated with the operational managers of the facilities where WBCHCWs were attached to and arranged with them on the date and time for data collection. The purpose of the study and the ethical issues were highlighted to the participants. Ward-based community health workers who consented to the study were included as participants.

2.5.2 Pilot study

Before data collection, a pilot study was conducted, which guided the researcher on how to conduct the main study in terms of framing the research question and the time needed to conduct the study. One FGD was conducted in one of the PHC facilities from the same sub-district, with five (5) participants in one (1) group having the same characteristics as the participants who participated in the main study. Participants were selected using purposive sampling, and their results were not included in the main study.

2.5.3 Process of data collection

The researcher used the FGD interview guide to collect data from the participants. Data was collected in the PHC facility where WBCHCWs were attached to. A hall was arranged where the researcher met with the participants, and it was conducted on various days, as three PHCs were used. One PHC had about 40 WBCHCWs who were allocated under the facility. The researcher collected data from the facility on different days. The groups were divided into 10 participants per FGD, bringing the total of four (4) who participated in the study. Data was collected using Sepedi as the dominant language spoken at Sekhukhune District. The researcher asked one central question which was *what challenges do you experience when using the diabetic and hypertension screening tool on patients in the community?* Participants were given time to process the question and were spontaneous in responding. Probing questions to obtain more detail and clarity on the participants' challenges were asked. The Ward Based Outreach Team Leaders of the three (3) PHC facilities were approached to be researchers' assistants in advance to assist in taking field notes. A voice recorder was used to record the interviews with the consent of the participants. The focus group discussion lasted for 40–45 minutes, and data was collected over 3 weeks between March and April 2022.

2.5.4 Data analysis

Thematic analysis was used to analyse the data as it involves the identification of themes, patterns, regularities, and inconsistencies [14]. Data was transcribed as stated by participants. The researcher repeatedly read the data actively while searching for meanings and patterns and taking notes for coding. Codes identify characteristics of the data that the researcher finds interesting. To do this, the researcher organized the data into meaningful groups. The codes were then sorted into different themes, and the relevant codes extracted within the themes were grouped. Relations between codes, themes, and sub-themes were identified. The themes were reviewed and refined and were analysed until they formed a coherent pattern. The validity of individual themes concerning the data was considered. The essence of what each theme captured was identified. Each theme was analysed in detail. Finally, three themes and six sub-themes emerged from the current study.

2.6 Measures to ensure trustworthiness

To ensure trustworthiness, credibility, transferability, conformability, and dependability were applied in this study [16]. The strategies to enhance credibility, which are prolonged engagement, persistent observation, and peer debriefing, were applied. The researcher invested enough time, established trust in the WBCHWs, kept the inquiry honest, and identified elements relevant to the study. In this study, the field notes and transcriptions were given to an independent coder who had not participated in the study to analyse and interpret. The transcribed data was handed to the supervisor to recheck and ensure that all findings are supported by data from the participants. Audit recordings were helpful as a part of the audit trail and also served as a reminder. The researcher provided enough information for the reader to determine if the findings were transferable to another context. Generalizing could not be considered in the study, as the study was limited to three PHC facilities in Limpopo province.

2.7 Ethical considerations

Ethical approval was obtained from the Research Committee of the Faculty of Health Sciences of the University of Pretoria, project number 167/2020, and the Department of Health Research Committee of Limpopo Province. The researcher also received permission from the District Executive, the assistant manager, and operational managers of the selected PHC facilities. Before commencing with the FDGs, participants were given leaflets with full information about the study, which was followed by verbal information. The researcher obtained voluntary written informed consent from participants, and they were not forced to participate in the study. To ensure anonymity, the names of three PHC facilities were referred to as facility 1, 2, and 3, and these allocations are known by the researcher only. All participants responded anonymously based on the code that corresponds to the participants. The true identity of participants corresponds to each code known by the researcher. The participants were informed about their rights and their right to ask questions. They were also informed that they can withdraw from the study at any stage. Emphasis was also made to participants to keep the information provided by them confidential from all the groups.

3. Results

From the collected data, three themes with six sub-themes were identified as indicated in **Table 1**.

3.1 Theme 1: Challenges experienced by WBCHWs regarding the utilization of non-communicable screening tools

Table 1 indicates the challenges experienced by participants as follows: WBCHWs-related challenges, which encompass the limited scope of practice and poor recognition; client-related challenges, which include inadequate cooperation with screening and distrust of WBCHWs by patients and family members; and resource-related challenges, which cover lack of screening tools and shortage of equipment. The themes and sub-themes are discussed below:

3.1.1 WBCHWs-related challenges

From this theme, two themes emerged as limited scope of practice and poor recognition. As a challenge, WBCHWs indicated that they know their scope of practice, although when they go for screening, they work beyond that. Ward-based community health workers reported that they are frustrated by the workload they are doing, and they are not recognized by the government for the work they do.

Themes	Sub-themes
WBCHW-related challenges	• Limited scope of practice • Poor recognition
Clients-related challenges	• Distrust by family members and the community • Inadequate cooperation from clients and family members
Resource-related challenges	• Lack of screening tools • Shortage of equipment

Table 1.
Main theme: Challenges experienced by WBCHCW.

3.1.1.1 Limited scope of practice

During the focus group discussion, some participants indicated that their scope of practice is limited. They reported that the EMS staff, when picking up patients that they referred, ask them for information that they know very well that it is above their scope of work, which they are not allowed to practice, because they do not perform certain activities due to the scope of practice.

> **FG2-P2:** *"The EMS ambulance will ask what the problem with the patient is, they even ask for the BP readings of the patient, and even the patient's diagnosis, which we do not know about and are not trained to do, we conduct household screening and other activities, like giving health education for the screened conditions".*

> **FG2-P7** *shared the same sentiments: "in other houses/homes, when we screen them when we start introducing ourselves, they will ask us if we have BP machines and scales, they also ask if we have treatment for headaches, so we tell them how we work. However, they also ask questions that need hospital answers, and it becomes difficult for us to screen them."*

Another participant added

> **FG3-p7** *"Yes, some will even ask you after screening about their diagnosis. From the screening question, we advise them on what to do if we see that they are at risk and refer them; apart from that, there is nothing we can do."*

3.1.1.2 Poor recognition by family members, community, and government

Participants reported that their work is not fully recognized by the people they provide health care to, especially if their screening is not backed up by the use of an apparatus such as a blood pressure and a glucometer machine. Some even reported poor recognition by the government as they are paid a lower salary.

> **FG1-P3:** *"...but sometimes we come across those who want devices that we can use to check them, for example, the BP machine and glucometer, that is when they will believe in our work. We screen when they are open, but because they are not the same, some prefer to see us having something in our pocket to show that he/she might be having diabetes."*

In addition, other participants mentioned that some of the family members are rude and undermining the work done by WBCHWs, and they prefer to consult other healthcare providers whom they feel are better than WBCHWs.

> **FG3-P9**: *"Sometimes when screening the community member, they say that they have their private doctors, when he/she get sick they will go to their private doctor, so I felt undermined as a community health worker because we are working for the government."*

Participants also reported that they are being paid a stipend, which does not cover their family's financial responsibilities. They indicated that they feel that the government does not recognize them and the work they are doing on a daily basis. They are earning little.

> **FG3-P2:** *"As a community health worker, I work too much because I am a counsellor. I give counselling to community members. I am also a teacher because children when I do the screening, they ask me questions on health issues, which requires me to help them. I am also a pharmacist; I distribute patients' medication at home. I am also a psychologist who solves problems of the community members, but after this workload, the government does not even recognise us. We are doing too much work for the community, and our salaries never increase. We always sign contracts and are not absorbed permanently, but the department wants to report every month."*

Other participants added by saying;

> **FG1-P5 & FG2-P3:** *Yes, we are doing a lot for the community and the government, but the pay is not equal to the work we do. We also work in hot weather, and sometimes we visit the patients when it is raining. our pay is small; we wish the government and consider us and increase our salaries.*

The information shared here suggests that the scope of work for WBCHWs needs to be clarified and congruent with the training provided and also to their salary, as they feel they are not recognized.

3.1.2 Client-related challenges

From this theme, two sub-themes emerged, where participants reported inadequate cooperation from clients and distrust from family members and the community. Participants reported that when utilizing non-communicable screening tools, patients withhold information. Sometimes they provide wrong information, refuse to respond to questions, refuse to provide personal information, refuse to be screened, and do not want to participate in the counseling sessions. The following quotes confirm challenges as reported by participants.

> **FG1-P11:** *"Patients sometimes do not want to give us information. You are busy screening a person he/she just denies some of the things, but you can see that what you are asking is there. Which means that they withhold information."*

> **FG2-P2:** … *"even though sometimes they lie to us, we have to ask them questions".*

3.1.2.1 Inadequate cooperation from patients and family members

Participants reported that when they use the screening tools, sometimes family members and patients do not cooperate with them, and they refuse to provide the information needed to complete the tools. One participant reported that family members sometimes refused to give important information about the head of the family as required in the screening tools. This was supported by the following quote:

> **FG3-P9:** *"The challenge I had when I was screening hypertension, household, and diabetes was the head of the family refusing to provide information, especially with the names of the head of the family, phone numbers, and ID number.*
>
> **FG3-P5** *yes, some of the household members would refuse to give us the ID number and the phone number, saying they are private details."*

Another participant concurred with the challenges of a lack of cooperation by indicating that members of the community go out when they see WHCHCWs entering their homes. Some do not want to give them an opportunity to screen even when they see that this person is having signs of either hypertension or diabetic mellitus. This report was supported by the following quote.

> **FG1-P6:** *"Most of the community members refuse to be screened when we enter their homes; they go out. Most of them are sick, even when I try to give them health education and counselling, they do not want to listen to us. They tell you that they have a medical aid membership. Thus, I can see that they are sick, but they deny the screening, especially the men, they are the ones who do not want to be screened."*

The unwillingness to share information by patients/community members made it difficult for the team to write a clean report about the patient's condition, as they hide some of the information during screening.

3.1.2.2 Distrust by family members and the community

Ward-based community health workers experience challenges from family members and the community, whereby they do not trust that they are entrusted with the screening of non-communicable diseases by the Department of Health. One participant reported that the family members suspect and confuse robbers when they approach households. Participants reported that there are instances when clients will run away when they see them coming. Some family members hide ill patients; some see them as a threat to spreading COVID-19. Some of the clients even verbalize that they do not see any benefit from the work conducted by WBCHWs. This report was supported by the following quotes:

> **FG1-P5***: "When we go there not having anything, saying we are sent by the department verbally, it is as if we are lying, we are there to rob or cheat them, and that we are only there just to get our payment through them. Many people say it is only through them that we are paid."*

Another participant added by saying that they are seen as threats by the community and family members, people who will disclose the patient's condition.

FG2-P6: *"Some of the challenges when we go to the households, for hypertension and diabetes screening, some families run inside their houses and they will say those who disclose about people's conditions have arrived, or when you get them at home they will say they are visitors, they don't want to see us and we can't enter their house without their consent."*

It was evident that family members and the community did not trust WBCHCs as some see them as robbers, people who do not keep confidential information privately.

3.1.3 Resource-related challenges

From this theme, two sub-themes emerged where participants reported non-availability of screening tools and shortage of equipment, as indicated in **Table 1** above.

3.1.3.1 Non-availability of screening tools

Participants reported that a shortage of screening tools affected their daily services as they could not screen their patients thoroughly. This results in the WBCHWs using their money to photocopy so that they can look professional and respected by the community and family members. Regarding a lack of stationery and shortage of the screening tools, the participants mentioned that:

FG3-P5: *"Another challenge we have is the shortage of screening tools, this makes our work difficult as we cannot work without screening tool".*

FG3-P1: *"To add to what participant 5 has said, the departments of health send us the screening tools to the phone, and they want us to use our money to print screening tools, it makes our work difficult because we don't have money to print the screening tools, that's why we use our notebooks".*

FG1-P11: *"so the time I do not have, it means work will not be able to move. It is a stationery problem."*

FG1-P6: *"I go back to what participant 11 has highlighted, it takes us back that our work seems to be of no value because of these papers. I mean the screening tools. They are the ones who give us dignity when working with them in the community. So, when you start removing papers from a notebook, it seems like you are not serious about your work."*

3.1.3.2 Shortage of equipment

The shortage of equipment was also included as a challenging experience. Participants reported that sometimes they do not have photocopy machines to copy the screening tools, which in turn had a negative impact on the screening. The participants highlighted the following:

FG-P11 & FG2-P3: *"We do not have a photocopy machine; we make copies of this screening tool by ourselves. This means that the day we do not have money, we will not use screening tools, and it limits our work, we only screen those five families because we don't have a photocopy machine."*

Other participants added and reported the use of notebooks to screen members of the family. One even indicated of the tool being sent through the phone.

> **FG3-P5:** *"Another challenge we have is the shortage of screening tools; our photocopy machine was broken. We use the notebooks while referring to the phone screening tools when screening the patients for household diabetes and hypertension."*

Drawing from the discussions in focus groups. It was also obvious that the WBCHWs are experiencing challenges related to the non-availability of screening tools and equipment, which had a detrimental effect as they could not work properly.

4. Discussion

The study's findings highlighted that WBCHWs face various challenges when using screening tools for non-communicable diseases. These include WBCHW-related challenges described as a limited scope of practice and a lack of recognition by both the health system and communities. Then, client-related challenges involve distrust by family members and the community, as well as inadequate cooperation from clients and family members. Lastly, resource-related challenges involve lack of screening tools and a shortage of equipment. Collectively, these issues hinder the effective implementation of NCD screening programs in the rural communities of Limpopo Province, South Africa.

4.1 WBCHW-related challenges

A significant challenge identified pertains to the limited scope of practice and poor recognition of WBCHWs. Although WBCHWs scope of work in South Africa is described [16], it is often narrowly defined, constraining their ability to operate effectively beyond basic healthcare provision. The restricted scope limits WBCHWs to basic tasks such as health education, household visits, and the provision of basic care or referrals. The set scope does not enable them to play a more integrated role in disease prevention, management, and health promotion activities, particularly for non-communicable diseases (NCDs). According to Kok et al. [17], many community health worker programs in low and middle-class countries struggle with role ambiguity, which leads to ineffective service delivery. In the South African context, WBCHWs are often perceived as laypersons with limited clinical authority, which negatively affects both their confidence and the trust they command in communities [16].

Such limitations in their mandate not only constrain the potential impact of WBCHWs but also create a disconnect between community health needs and service provision. For instance, many rural communities face a rising burden of NCDs such as hypertension and diabetes, which require early detection, regular monitoring, and sustained lifestyle counseling services that WBCHWs could potentially offer if their roles were expanded and more clearly defined [17].

The lack of clarity around the WBCHWs' scope of work also impacts their acceptance within the broader health system. According to Schneider et al. [16], ambiguity in role definition often leads to poor integration of community health workers into primary healthcare teams, resulting in limited support, inadequate supervision, and low morale among WBCHWs. This, in turn, diminishes their effectiveness and undermines the sustainability of community-based health initiatives. In sum, the narrowly defined scope limits WBCHWs' ability to address the evolving health needs of rural populations effectively.

Furthermore, poor recognition by other health professionals and the community can be demoralizing and reduce the motivation of WBCHWs [18]. Scott et al. [16] highlight that for CHWs to be effective, they need not only technical skills but also social legitimacy and recognition from both the healthcare system and the community they serve. Without adequate support and acknowledgment, WBCHWs may experience burnout, diminished job satisfaction, and attrition.

Expanding and formalizing the scope of practice for WBCHWs through clear policies, adequate training, and integration into the health system can strengthen their ability to deliver care. This approach would enhance their contribution to addressing the dual burden of communicable and non-communicable diseases in underserved communities. In turn WBCHWs will be well recognized by the clients, family members, and community at large.

4.2 Client-related challenges

Two sub-themes emerged from the client-related challenges as inadequate cooperation with screening and distrust by family members and the broader community. These factors significantly hinder the uptake and effectiveness of non-communicable disease (NCD) screening services in rural communities. Firstly, inadequate cooperation with screening refers to instances where clients are unwilling or reluctant to participate in health assessments conducted by WBCHWs [19]. This can stem from a lack of awareness about the importance of screening, fear of being diagnosed with a chronic illness, or misconceptions about the purpose of the visit. Research by Meherali et al. [20] emphasizes that low health literacy in many low and middle-class communities' limits understanding of NCDs and the value of early detection, resulting in poor engagement with screening efforts. Additionally, some clients prioritize immediate, visible health issues over preventive care, viewing screening as unnecessary if they do not feel ill.

The success of NCD screening is heavily dependent on client engagement and cooperation. However, this study found that WBCHWs often encounter resistance or apathy from clients during household visits. Distrust by family members and the broader community is a serious barrier. Family and community members may be reluctant to engage with WBCHWs due to concerns about confidentiality, skepticism regarding the WBCHWs' competence, or cultural beliefs that conflict with biomedical approaches [17].

Distrust erodes the essential relationship between healthcare providers and clients, ultimately compromising the effectiveness of health interventions [21]. Many WBCHWs live in the same communities they serve, which can raise concerns about privacy and confidentiality. Community members may fear that personal health information will be shared informally, leading to stigma or gossip [22]. In a study by Munshi et al. [23], the role of trust was identified as pivotal in promoting community engagement with WBCHWs. Without trust, clients are less likely to disclose accurate information or follow health advice. In some cases, clients may question the qualifications of WBCHWs, perceiving them as less competent than clinic-based professionals, which further fuels mistrust. Where this trust is lacking, uptake of services such as NCD screening diminishes significantly.

Together, these sub-themes show that social and cultural dynamics play a crucial role in the success of health interventions. Addressing them requires more than clinical training, it demands targeted community engagement, health education campaigns, and efforts to build and maintain trust between WBCHWs and the populations they serve.

4.3 Resource-related challenges

The availability of screening tools and medical equipment is foundational to the WBCHWs' ability to conduct effective NCD assessments. Participants in this study reported frequent shortages of screening tools and equipment, which hampers their efficiency and credibility. The lack of glucometers, blood pressure monitors, and other essential tools renders WBCHWs powerless in identifying and managing conditions such as hypertension and diabetes at the community level.

Strengthening primary healthcare systems depends not only on human resources but also on the consistent availability of essential equipment, medical supplies, and robust information systems. Without these, even well-trained and motivated WBCHWs cannot fulfill their responsibilities effectively. The shortage of screening tools and equipment is a major barrier that undermines the ability of WBCHWs to deliver effective non-communicable disease (NCD) screening services in rural areas [24]. Moreover, logistical and supply chain constraints are among the biggest barriers to effective NCD management in rural settings. The WBCHWs assist the primary healthcare system to function well [25, 26], but the lack of resources affects their ability to screen effectively and damages their credibility in the eyes of the community, further reducing trust and service uptake. While WBCHWs are tasked with promoting health and detecting illness at the household level, their efforts are often compromised by inadequate tools and logistical support.

In summary, the lack of screening tools and equipment represents a structural weakness in the implementation of community-based NCD screening programs. It limits the efficiency of WBCHWs and contributes to the continued burden of undiagnosed or poorly managed chronic conditions in rural South Africa. Ensuring consistent supply chains and investment in essential tools is therefore critical for the success of primary healthcare interventions.

5. Conclusion

The results of this study highlighted the challenges experienced by WBCHWs regarding the utilization of non-communicable screening tools and were related to a limited scope of practice and recognition. The findings of this study indicated that a shortage of screening tools and equipment causes distrust towards WBCHWs and inadequate cooperation with the screening of family members in the households. Despite the shortage of resources, WBCHWs compensate for the screening services by using their money to print the screening tools. As such, the provision of sufficient resources, a clear scope of practice, recognition of WBCHWs by both the community and government, and capacitation of WBCHWs will improve their working conditions; hence addressing Sustainable Development Goal number 3 of good health to all and reduction of non-communicable diseases of service.

6. Study limitation

The findings of this study cannot be generalized to other provinces as the study was limited to three clinics in Limpopo Province. The study was not funded; hence, the researcher used her resources to conduct the research, which limited the study setting.

Acknowledgements

Researchers would like to thank EM who was involved in the conceptualization of the study, all the WBCHWs who participated in the study, and the Limpopo Department of Health, who gave permission for this study to be conducted.

Author contribution

TIR and MMR were involved in the conceptualization of the study, drafting of this paper, and its finalization.

Conflict of interest

There is no conflict of interest regarding the publication of this paper.

Data availability statement

Supporting data for the findings of this research is available on request.

Author details

Irene Ramavhoya Thifhelimbilu* and Melitah Rasweswe Molatelo
Department of Nursing Science, University of Limpopo, Sovenga, South Africa

*Address all correspondence to: irene.ramavhoya@ul.ac.za

References

[1] Bouvard V, Wentzensen N, Mackie A, Berkhof J, Brotherton J, Giorgi-Rossi P, et al. The IARC perspective on cervical cancer screening. New England Journal of Medicine. 2021;**385**(20):1908-1918

[2] Malau E, Ramavhoya IT, Rasweswe MM. Importance of utilizing non-communicable disease screening tools; ward-based community health care workers of South Africa explain. International Journal of Environmental Research and Public Health. 2024;**21**(3):263

[3] World Health Organization. Global Status Report on Noncommunicable Diseases. Geneva, Switzerland: WHO Library Cataloguing-in-Publication Data; World Health Organization; 2010. Available from: http://www.who.int [Accessed: April 12, 2025]

[4] Mhlongo EM, Lutge E. The roles, responsibilities, and perceptions of community health workers and ward-based primary health care outreach teams (WBPHCOTs) in South Africa: A scoping review protocol. Systematic Reviews. 2019;**8**:193

[5] Elelwani M. Experiences of ward-based community health care workers regarding the utilisation of patients screening tools in Fetakgomo-Tubatse Subdistrict, Limpopo Province [Master's thesis]. Pretoria, South Africa: University of Pretoria; 2022

[6] World Health Organization (WHO). Adapting the WHO Package of Essential Non-communicable Diseases Interventions. Vol. 96. Netherlands: Department of Health Promotion, Faculty of Health, Maastricht University; 2018. pp. 578-583

[7] Goh YS, Ow Yong QYJ, Soo SC, Wan PCJ, Ng VCK. Experiences and challenges faced by community mental health workers when providing care to people with mental health conditions: A qualitative descriptive study. International Journal of Mental Health Nursing. 2022;**31**(3):591-600

[8] Johnson LJ, Schopp LH, Waggie F, Frantz JM. Challenges experienced by community health workers and their motivation to attend a self-management programme. African Journal of Primary Health Care & Family Medicine. 2022;**14**(1):2911

[9] Salve S, Raven J, Das P, Srinivasan S, Khaled A, Hayee M, et al. Community health workers and Covid-19: Cross-country evidence on their roles, experiences, challenges and adaptive strategies. PLOS Global Public Health. 2023;**3**(1):e0001447

[10] Tshitangano TG, Olaniyi FC. Sustaining the national health insurance scheme in South Africa: The roles and challenges of community health workers. The Open Public Health Journal. 2018;**11**(1):494-506

[11] Jobson G, Naidoo N, Matlakala N, Marincowitz G, Railton J, McIntyre JA, et al. Contextual factors affecting the integration of community health workers into the health system in Limpopo Province, South Africa. International Health. 2020;**12**(4):281-286

[12] Census. Municipal Report. Polokwane, South Africa, Limpopo: Limpopo Statistics; 2023. Available from: https://www.statssa.gov.za/ [Accessed: January 12, 2024]

[13] Brink H, Van der Walt C. Fundamentals of Research Methodology

for Health Care Professionals. Cape Town, South Africa: Juta and Company Ltd.; 2022

[14] Polit DF, Beck CT. Essentials of Nursing Research: Appraising Evidence for Nursing Practice. 10th ed. Philadelphia: Wolters Kluwer; 2022

[15] Barrett D, Twycross A. Data Collection in Qualitative Research, Evidence-Based Nursing. 7th ed Vol. 21(3). Ghana: Rose Marie Bailey; 2018. pp. 63-64

[16] Schneider H, Besada D, Daviaud E, Sanders D, Rohde S. Ward-based primary health care outreach teams in South Africa: Developments, challenges and future directions. South African Health Review. 2018;**2018**:59-65.9

[17] Kok MC, Dieleman M, Taegtmeyer M, Broerse JE, Kane SS, Ormel H, et al. Which intervention design factors influence the performance of community health workers in low- and middle-income countries? A systematic review. Health Policy and Planning. 2015;**30**(9):1207-1227. DOI: 10.1093/heapol/czu126

[18] Singh P. One Million Community Health Workers: Global Technical Taskforce Report. New York: The Earth Institute, Columbia University; 2013. Available from: http://1millionhealthworkers.org/files/2013/01/1mCHW_TechnicalTaskForceReport.pdf

[19] Le Bonniec A, Sun S, Andrin A, Dima AL, Letrilliart L. Barriers and facilitators to participation in health screening: An umbrella review across conditions. Prevention Science. 2022;**23**:1115-1142. DOI: 10.1007/s11121-022-01388-y

[20] Meherali S, Punjani NS, Mevawala A. Health literacy interventions to improve health outcomes in low- and middle-income countries. Health Literacy Research and Practice. 2020;**4**(4):e251-e266. DOI: 10.3928/24748307-20201118-01

[21] Scott K, Beckham SW, Gross M, Pariyo G, Rao KD, Cometto G, et al. What do we know about community-based health worker programs? A systematic review of existing reviews on community health workers. Human Resources for Health. 2018;**16**(1):39. DOI: 10.1186/s12960-018-0304-x

[22] Jobson G, Naidoo N, Matlakala N, Marincowitzc G, Railtona J, McIntyre JA, et al. Contextual factors affecting the integration of community health workers into the health system in Limpopo Province, South Africa. International Health. 2020;**12**:281-286. DOI: 10.1093/inthealth/ihz082

[23] Munshi S, Christofides NJ, Eyles J. Sub-national perspectives on the implementation of a national community health worker programme in Gauteng Province, South Africa. BMJ Global Health. 2019;**4**(Suppl. 10):e001564. DOI: 10.1136/bmjgh-2019-001564

[24] Marcus TS, Hugo J, Jinabhai CC. Which primary care model? A qualitative analysis of ward-based outreach teams in South Africa. African Journal of Primary Health Care & Family Medicine. 2017;**9**(1):a1252. DOI: 10.4102/phcfm.v9i1.1252

[25] Assegaai T, Reagon G, Schneider H. Evaluating the effect of ward-based outreach teams on primary healthcare performance in Northwest Province, South Africa: A plausibility design using routine data. South African Medical Journal. 2018;**108**(4):329-335. DOI: 10.7196/SAMJ. 2018.v108i4.12755

[26] Assegaai T, Schneider H. Factors associated with workplace and interpersonal trust in the supervisory system of a community health worker programme in a rural South African District. International Journal of Health Policy and Management. 2021;**11**(1):1-8. DOI: 10.34172/ijhpm.2021.03

Section 3

Community-Based and Workforce Perspectives in Primary Care

Chapter 5

The Impact of COVID-19 on Primary Health Care-Seeking Behaviour: Voices of Learner Nurses from a Selected University in Limpopo Province, South Africa

Takalani Edith Mutshatshi

Abstract

The outbreak of COVID-19 has affected the primary health care-seeking behavior of all citizens, including learner nurses. The health-seeking behavior amongst learner nurses at a university in Limpopo Province has decreased greatly during the COVID-19 pandemic. The study aimed to investigate the impact of COVID-19 on health-seeking behavior as voiced by the learner nurses from a university in Limpopo, South Africa. A qualitative, explorative, and descriptive design was used. A non-probability purposive sampling method was used. Data was collected through semi-structured interviews, saturated at the 12th participant, analyzed using Tesch's open coding method, and the themes and sub-themes were developed. The key findings of the study revealed that learner nurses were afraid to visit primary health care (PHC) centres for fear of infection and lack of information versus myths related to COVID-19, and suggestions were identified to improve health-seeking behavior during the COVID-19 pandemic. The study recommends knowledge empowerment of the community during pandemics to improve primary health-seeking behavior in health care institutions.

Keywords: impact, primary health care, health-seeking behavior, learner nurse, COVID-19

1. Introduction

Primary health care-seeking behavior is a global challenge experienced by individuals, commonly noted during the post-pandemic eruption due to fear and uncertainty. This health-seeking behavior refers to any measure that an individual undertakes after perceiving themselves to have a health problem or illness to find a better or appropriate remedy in any primary health care setting, with some seeking such health-related information over the internet [1, 2]. The study conducted by Tran and Silvestri-Elmore [3] revealed that the current body of knowledge related to

 IntechOpen

health care-seeking behavior, the utilization of health information resources, and its impact on health care-seeking behavior and barriers to accessing care amongst this population is still a major challenge.

Primary health care (PHC) is an important mode of health service believed to be the basis of the health service pyramid, as it involves providing continuous, comprehensive health services, which include preventive and curative health services [4]. Furthermore, health care-seeking behavior is any action or inaction undertaken by individuals who perceive themselves to have a health problem or to be ill to find an appropriate remedy [5]. When seeking health, a person may turn to conventional healers or self-medication [6]. Furthermore, it confirms that before the outbreak of COVID-19, there was a decrease in health-seeking behavior, although in small percentages due to other personal reasons, but with the emergence of the COVID-19 pandemic, there was a swift increase, where people were reluctant to visit health care institutions [6].

The outbreak of COVID-19 worldwide has affected the primary health care-seeking behavior of all citizens in primary health settings, including the learners at different institutions of higher learning. People lost the courage to visit the primary health care facilities when they had sickness symptoms; instead, they consulted family and friends to get their medications from health workers in the pharmacy [7]. This is due to fear of stigma towards them should they test positive and fear of having their whole family and friends get transferred into quarantine or having to disclose their activities for contact tracing. Some other factors for not seeking medical help are the responsibility of the family, the fear of isolation by society, the fear of breaking off a relationship, social stigma, and a lack of societal support [8].

The evidence from countries like Ethiopia, which had a previous epidemic, reveals that people tend to lose trust in the primary health care system and have a fear of developing a disease in the health facility. Therefore, they decided to avoid seeking treatment for their illness or sending a loved one for medical care, leading to an increased mortality rate from their previous illnesses, not COVID-19. Therefore, this outbreak led to a decrease in the number of hospital visits. For example, in pediatric outpatient and chronic care clinics, hospital visits dropped by 30–70% in April 2020 [9].

In a survey conducted in South Africa, 60.1% of respondents reported that they were concerned about the impact of COVID-19 on their health since the lockdown in South Africa on 27 March 2020, and 98.1% of them reported that they had changed their behavior by only leaving the house to buy essentials [10]. Around 43.8% reported that they visited the pharmacy once or twice, and 54% indicated that they would not seek health care because they fear getting infected in the health care facility. Thus, it is along this background that the study seeks to explore and describe the impact of COVID-19 on the primary health care-seeking behavior of learner nurses at a university in Limpopo Province, South Africa [10].

2. Clarification of the key concepts

The key concepts that are in use in this chapter are clarified in detail below to increase understanding of the aspects.

2.1 Impact

The change that occurs in someone or something, caused by someone or something, resulting in noticeable negative consequences [11]. In this study, the impact is the after-effects of COVID-19 on the primary health care-seeking behavior of learner nurses at a university in South Africa, subsequently decreasing the utilization of such services.

2.2 COVID-19

COVID-19 is the name given by the World Health Organization in 2020 for the disease caused by the SARS-CoV-2 coronavirus, which started in Wuhan (China) in late 2019 [12]. In this study, COVID-19 refers to the disease outbreak that started in 2019 and ended up affecting the whole globe, impacting the health-seeking behavior of communities, including learners at institutions of higher learning.

2.3 Learner nurse

A learner nurse is a person undergoing education and training in nursing and must be registered with the South African Nursing Council [13]. In this study, a learner nurse is a student registered with the Department of Nursing Science at a university in Limpopo Province whose primary health care-seeking behavior is affected by the COVID-19 pandemic.

2.4 Health

The World Health Organization [12] defined health as complete physical, mental, and social well-being in the absence of any disease or impairment that allows the individual to adequately cope with the demands of daily life. In this study, health refers to the ability of learner nurses to survive any disease, being free from illness (spiritual, physical, and mental), thus meeting the goals for survival.

2.5 Behavior

Behavior is a range of actions and mannerisms made by individuals [14]. In this study, behavior is the way learner nurses take action to attend to their health needs during the COVID-19 pandemic.

2.6 Primary health care (PHC)

Refers to essential health care that is based on "scientifically sound and socially acceptable methods and technology, which make universal health care accessible to all individuals and families in a community" (Declaration of Alma–Ata, 1978 & [15]). In the study, PHC refers to the first level of contact in seeking health care, where, in this study, the learner nurses were to seek health care during the COVID-19 pandemic.

3. Research methods

3.1 Research approach and design

The study followed a qualitative approach to collect data from learner nurses on their views on primary health care-seeking behavior during the COVID-19 pandemic, and this approach enabled the researcher to obtain in-depth information. The study adopted a qualitative, explorative, and descriptive research design to explore and describe the health care-seeking behavior of learner nurses during COVID-19.

3.2 Population, sampling, and sample size

The population was all registered learner nurses in their third and fourth years of study, and a total of 140 learner nurses. Selection of participants employed a non-probability purposive heterogeneous sampling method with a predetermined inclusion criterion. The sample size was determined by data saturation when no new information emerged at participant 14.

3.3 Data collection and analysis

A semi-structured face-to-face interview, with an interview guide, was used to obtain data from participants until data saturation at participant 14. A voice recorder was used to capture data as per permission granted by participants, with additional field notes to capture the non-verbal cues. The duration of the interview session took 20–45 minutes. Data audio recorded and field notes were then transcribed verbatim. Analysis of the data was conducted using Tesch's open coding method to develop themes and sub-themes, with the involvement of an independent coder, where consensus on themes and sub-themes was reached.

4. Results

The data was collected from 14 participants, all registered students, including six third-year and eight fourth-year nursing students at a selected university in Limpopo Province. The participants were predominantly female, reflecting the long-standing trend of nursing as a female-dominated profession. The demographic profile featured eight female nursing students and six male students, all aged 20–23 (**Table 1**).

Themes	Sub-themes
1. Fear of infection	1. Infection during consultation 2. Stigma on diagnosis of COVID-19 3. Fear of undergoing quarantine, hospitalization, and death
2. Lack of information versus myths related to COVID-19	1. Inadequate knowledge and information on COVID-19 2. False information about prevention, spread, and treatment of COVID-19
3. Suggestions to improve health-seeking behavior during COVID-19	1. The use of advanced technology for consultation during pandemics 2. Health education to the community 3. Provision of adequate equipment and supplies

Table 1.
Represents the themes and sub-themes that originate from the study.

4.1 Fear of infection

The study findings exposed that there is a fear of infection amongst learner nurses. Below is a detailed explanation of the identified sub-themes: fear of being infected during consultation, stigma attached to the diagnosis, and prolonged waiting times in the primary health care facilities.

4.1.1 Infection during consultation

The findings of the study revealed that learner nurses were afraid to visit the health facilities for consultation due to the fear that they could be infected with COVID-19. The learner nurses were also afraid to be assessed and diagnosed with COVID-19 if they visited the health care facilities. This finding is evidenced by the following quotes:

Another participant, participant 5, said, *"As a student, I became very scared of going to the health care facilities to seek services, because I was afraid of contracting COVID-19."*

Furthermore, another participant, participant 7, said, *"I became scared because I was afraid that if I consult, I'll end up contracting the virus. I would go to pharmacy to get the type of medication that I want whenever I was sick."*

4.1.2 Stigma on diagnosis of COVID-19

The findings of this study found that learner nurses have a fear of being stigmatized if they are diagnosed with COVID-19, which prevents learner nurses from consulting primary health care during the COVID-19 pandemic. The findings further indicated that if a learner nurse goes to the health facility, they are already labeled as having COVID-19, and in turn, they present with fear of being stigmatized. The findings are supported by the following quotes:

Participant 3: "*The stigma of being tested positive because when you test positive for COVID-19 A lot of people stigmatize you and they end up not wanting to be in contact with you and they might isolate you and that will cause me to overthink that I will die from COVID-19.*"

Participant 6: "*The media, the stigma, that was attached to COVID-19 makes us fear to consult.*"

Participant 9 added that "I *had fear to go to consult because I feared that they would test me for COVID. If I test positive, I was afraid that I will be labeled as having Covid and I did not like that at all.*"

4.1.3 Fear of undergoing quarantine, hospitalization, and death

The findings of the study revealed that there was no way the health care providers would let a person go if they had symptoms of COVID-19 or had tested positive. People were put into quarantine for 14 days, which is very long. The findings revealed that learner nurses had a fear of undergoing the quarantine period and hospitalization and death due to COVID-19.

"*After 14 days they discharged me, ever since that I have never consulted during the pandemic because I was afraid of contracting the virus and being hospitalized again,*" reported participant 8.

"*It has affected me negatively because before COVID-19 I would go to the health care facility to consult for any illness that I had. Whereas during COVID-19 I was afraid to go to consult because I feared that they would test me for COVID,*" added participant 9.

4.2 Lack of information versus myths related to COVID-19

The findings of the study discovered that there is inadequate knowledge and information on COVID-19 and false information about the prevention, spread, and treatment of COVID-19.

4.2.1 Inadequate knowledge and information on COVID-19

The findings of the study revealed that a lack of knowledge about COVID-19 resulted in a lot of people having a misconception about COVID-19 and not visiting the hospital as they used to.

Participant 5 reported that "*lack of information about the condition, as it was a new virus to all so no one had experience in dealing with the infection*".

Participant 6 reported that "*The media and the stigma, that was attached to COVID-19 makes us fear to consult and this was due to lack of correct information people get from others.*"

4.2.2 False information about prevention, spread, and treatment of COVID-19

The findings of the study revealed that to gain publicity, people and companies formed lies about the virus not being there and told people to relax. Other people and companies increased the citizens' anxieties about COVID-19. People had a fear of consulting because they did not know what to believe. Therefore, they would rather stay at home and die or take care of themselves. Because of these misconceptions, people did not follow instructions at all.

Participant 6 said, "*For me generally, I was filled with a lot of fear. When I wanted to go seek health care, I had a lot of fear because as we all knew COVID-19 had some myths attached to it.*"

Participant 9 reported that "*The stigma of being tested positive because when you test positive for COVID-19 A lot of people stigmatize you as that person who tested positive you end up they end up not wanting to be in contact with you.*"

4.3 Suggestions to improve health-seeking behavior during pandemics

The findings of the study suggest that primary health care-seeking behavior can be improved by the use of advanced technology for consultation during pandemics, providing health education to people about COVID-19 to improve knowledge, and providing adequate equipment and supplies to control the spread of COVID-19 infection.

4.3.1 The use of advanced technology for consultation

People were advised to make appointments with the health facility because if they failed to do so, no attention would be given to the patient. This was done to manage the number of people coming to the health facility to prevent overcrowding or congestion, as it could lead to COVID-19 spreading more easily.

"*It was so difficult for us, maybe if the consultation was digital, it would be better like telemedicine that we read of, I mean using technology in 9health care as times go with technology,*" *said* participant 9.

"*So, before COVID-19 things were easier, we could easily access the health care facilities for help but during COVID-19 we were expected to book for a consultation in the university's health care centre, which affected us negatively because sometimes when you book, your consultation time or date might be tomorrow or later during the day which inconveniences you because you might be needing help at the moment,*" said participant 11.

4.3.2 Health education to the community

The finding revealed that other students were afraid of contracting the virus due to a lack of information. It is supported by participant no. 5, who stated that "*As a student, I became very scared of going to the health care facilities to seek their services, because I was afraid of contracting COVID-19.*"

Participant 5 suggested that "*the department of health, together with all the universities, should provide the information to all the students so that they will be very knowledgeable about the condition and how to prevent the infection.*"

And participant 2 suggested that "*People must be educated to have more information.*"

4.3.3 Provision of adequate equipment and supplies

Providing personal protective clothing can help decrease the fear and anxiety that people have about COVID-19 and improve their health-seeking behaviors. Participant 6 suggested that "the government should have provided more personal protective equipments (PPEs) to the public, and then they will generally go to the primary health care to seek health care."

Participant 8 suggested that "*but I think it'd have been better if the people who consult were also given PPE when they consult, so that they do not go with the virus at home because I think that the virus is everywhere, and you can take it home by your clothes.*"

Participant 7 suggested that "*Yeah, they should have tasked the home-based care nurses to go around testing people at home.*"

4.4 Discussion of findings

The findings of this study regarding fear to get infected during consultation are supported by another study conducted by Yousefi *et al.* [16, 17], which indicated that the flow of people in hospitals during the Covid pandemic brought along not only decreased numbers of non-emergency patients consulting but also the reduction for the emergency patients also consulting for fear of the COVID-19 infection. Furthermore, this finding also displays that clients' primary health care seeking behaviors heal have changed slightly in the emergence of the COVID-19 pandemic. According to Kugelman *et al.* [18], the COVID-19 outbreak caused much fear, leading people to be reluctant to seek medical care due to fear of contracting the infection.

The study findings further correspond to another study's findings, where the existence of significant stigma amongst COVID-19 patients makes them isolated, and this was evidenced by growing cases of stigma and discrimination in some societies and population groups for suffering from COVID-19 [19]. There is also an increased fear of stigma, where people also avoid screening, as stigmatized people are vulnerable to social avoidance and poor health-seeking behavior, leading to denial of patient admission in hospitals in Uganda [20]. The fear of isolation, admission, and death is highlighted in the study conducted by Jamili *et al.* [21], concluding that patients with COVID-19 experience stress, fear, and concerns in the course of their disease while hospitalized. Furthermore, the study recommends that a greater insight into patients' experiences is imperative to effectively address the disease, together with the provision of nursing care and psychological services. Another study's findings by Alipour *et al.* [22] also alluded to clients' experience of fear and stress from hospitalization and death from COVID-19, hence suggesting a need for psychological distress intervention.

The findings on inadequate knowledge of COVID-19 are supported by a study conducted by Schmidt *et al.* [23], revealing that false information circulated on social media not only instigated confusion, fear, and panic but also contributed to the creation of misconceptions and stigmatizing responses to COVID-19. According to Tedros [24], approximately 6000 people around the globe were hospitalized due to coronavirus misinformation. The misinformation on COVID-19 increases the fear and anxiety of people visiting primary health care facilities. According to Freeman *et al.* [25], the findings also conclude that there is a relationship between belief in COVID-19 conspiracies and an increase in vaccine uncertainty, like the belief that the virus is bioengineered, and therefore the people were less likely to report compliance with public health guidelines, and this contributed to reluctance in accepting the COVID-19 vaccine. Furthermore, another study by Gisondi *et al.* [26] also confirmed that COVID-19 was classified as the third leading cause of death in the United States, where the unvaccinated people continue to die in high numbers. Vaccine hesitancy and vaccine refusal were fuelled by COVID-19 misinformation and disinformation on social media platforms.

During pandemics like COVID-19, primary health institutions were deemed not to be effectively using technology to manage the pandemic and control the spread; hence, the study findings recommend improved utilization of technology. According to O'Brien and McNicholas [27], since the outbreak, the primary consideration has been one of safety and adherence to mandated physical distancing measures. Telemedicine is regarded as another means to provide a means to bring doctors and patients together without risking contamination. With regard to suspected cases of COVID-19, this approach to primary health care allows for triage without health care worker exposure to the virus. Telemedicine holds promise for future use, as it rationalizes human resources and reduces patient contact and thus infection risks [28].

The suggested intervention from the current study to effectively manage the pandemic was the education and empowerment of the community structures on COVID-19 issues, which seemed inadequate. The reason behind his statement was a lack of information about the virus; this means that students had only a fear of contracting the virus without knowing the background of the virus, such as the virus on its own, causative factors, how it is spread, preventive measures, medical management of the virus, and home management of the virus, etc. [29]. According to Lüdecke and Von Dem Knesebeck [29], disease-specific knowledge is essential to enable people to judge information on COVID-19. Health education programmes aimed at improving COVID-19 knowledge help shape appropriate practices and reduce the spread of the disease. Intervention strategies are thus needed to ensure easy access and better dissemination of high-quality information to the public.

Inadequate resources, both human and material, were revealed to be the major cause of poor primary health-seeking behavior, and the study recommends sufficient resource allocation for primary health care settings. A significant concern during the COVID-19 pandemic was the shortage of personal protective equipment, which increased pressure on health care workers and placed the community at risk of infection [30]. The shortages of personal protective equipment then led to improvisation and makeshift solutions. A study in the UK concluded that if health care workers had consistently received personal protective equipment, along with training in its use and extensive supervision and support from the government, they could have continued to provide and receive care effectively [30].

4.5 Limitations of the study

The study was limited to the selected university in Limpopo Province, in terms of the population, and used purposive sampling, so the findings may not be generalized to all other universities in Limpopo Province and South African universities at large. Other learner nurses in different institutions could have possibly generated different views and experiences.

4.6 Implications for policy, nursing, education, and health care preparedness

The findings of the current study may benefit the following:

- Policymakers

  The findings may inform policymakers on the need to develop effective policies regarding effective management of pandemics to ensure effective utilization of services, and where policies exist, the findings may inform policymakers to review the available policies to align them with the current disease and infection trend for successful management of future pandemics.

- Nursing practice and health care preparedness

  The findings of the study may assist nursing practice in redesigning patient care strategies to improve service delivery, especially in times of pandemic, and to improve infection control strategies in nursing practice so that nursing practice is kept abreast and fully prepared to deal with possible future pandemics.

- Nursing education and training

  The findings will inform nursing education institutions to be proactive and plan how to address future pandemic situations that may impact students' teaching and learning and primary health care, as well as to include effective infection control strategies during curriculum development, teaching, and learning in light of possible future pandemics.

4.7 Recommendations for future research

The study findings may prompt other researchers to explore further issues of preparedness for effective management of possible pandemics in the future, evaluation of the lessons learnt from the COVID-19 pandemic, and improvement on the gaps learnt from the pandemic. The study recommends that other researchers explore more on infection control-related issues, patient care delivery, and improvement plans for possible pandemics that may erupt in the future.

5. Conclusions

Primary health care-seeking behavior remains a challenge during pandemics, and this requires interventive strategies aimed at addressing the challenge to reduce mortality and morbidity in the entire community. This chapter covered the introduction, the clarification of concepts used in the chapter, and the methodology used, which relates to the research approach, the design, the population, sampling, sample size, data collection, and data analysis methods. Furthermore, the presentation, interpretation, and discussion of the findings on the impact of primary health care-seeking behavior during the COVID-19 pandemic were discussed in detail. Challenges such as a fear of infection, stigma attached, and long waiting times. Lack of information, shortage of material resources, lack of knowledge and skills, and some suggestions to improve primary health care-seeking behavior amongst learner nurses during pandemics.

Acknowledgements

The author would like to acknowledge the undergraduate students from a university in Limpopo Province. South African learner nurses who agreed to participate in the study.

Funding

There was no funding received for conducting the study.

Conflict of interest

The authors declare no conflict of interest.

Ethical approval

The study received ethical clearance from the Turfloop Research Ethics Committee (TREC/313/2022:UG).

Author details

Takalani Edith Mutshatshi
University of Limpopo Department of Nursing Science, Polokwane, South Africa

*Address all correspondence to: takalani.mutshatshi@ul.ac.za

References

[1] Afolabi MO, Irinoye A, Adegoke AA. Health-Seeking Behaviour and Student Perception of Health Care Services in a University Community in Nigeria. Pretoria, South Africa: Scientific Research Publishing; 2013

[2] Ahmad A, Khan MN, Rahman O. Exploring the use of the internet by university students for seeking health-related information. Interactive Technology and Smart Education. 2017;**14**(4):279-295

[3] Tran DMT, Silvestri-Elmore A. Healthcare-seeking behaviours in college students and young adults: A review. Journal of Research in Nursing. 2021;**26**(4):320-338

[4] Çakmur H. Introductory chapter: Why primary health care is essential? In: Primary Care Medicine-Theory and Practice. London, UK: IntechOpen; 2024

[5] Latunji OO, Akinyemi OO. Factors influencing health-seeking behaviour among civil servants in Ibadan, Nigeria. Annals of Ibadan Postgraduate Medicine. 2018;**16**(1):52-60

[6] Khadka S, Shrestha O, Koirala G, Acharya U, Adhikari G. Health seeking behavior and self-medication practice among undergraduate medical students of a teaching hospital: A cross-sectional study. Annals of Medicine and Surgery. 2022;**78**:103776

[7] Tran BX, Vu GT, Latkin CA, Pham HQ, Phan HT, Le HT, et al. Characterize the health and economic vulnerabilities of workers to control the emergence of COVID-19 in an industrial zone in Vietnam. Safety Science. 2020;**129**:104811

[8] Arti SS, Gandhar SS. A cross sectional study to assess the willingness and hesitancy regarding COVID-19 vaccination. Journal of Cardiovascular Disease Research. 2021;**12**(4):486-494

[9] Tamirat KS, Tessema ZT, Kebede FB. Factors associated with perceived barriers of health care access among reproductive-age women in Ethiopia: A secondary data analysis of 2016 Ethiopian demographic and health survey. BMC Health Services Research. 2020;**20**:1-8

[10] Statistic South Africa. Behavioural and Health Impacts of the COVID-19 Pandemic in South Africa. Pretoria, South Africa; 2020

[11] Murray JAH. Oxford Advanced Learner's Dictionary of Current English Oxford Sv Context. 8th ed. Oxford University Press; 2015

[12] World Health Organization. Rolling Updates on Coronavirus Disease (COVID-19). Geneva: World Health Organization; 2020

[13] Republic of South Africa. The Nursing Act, Act No. 33 of 2005 as Amended. Pretoria: Government Printer; 2008

[14] Longbing. In-depth behaviour understanding: The behaviour informatics approach. Information Science. 2010;**180**(17):3067-3085

[15] World Health Organization. Declaration of Alma-Ata 1978 Conference. Alma-Ata: Union of Soviet Socialist Republic; 2015

[16] Yousefi M, Yousefi M, Fathi M, Fogliatto FS. Patient visit forecasting in an emergency department using a deep neural network approach. Kybernetes. 2020;**49**(9):2335-2348

[17] Yucesan M et al. A forecasting model for patient arrivals of an emergency department in healthcare management systems. In: Intelligent Systems for Healthcare Management and Delivery. 2019

[18] Kugelman N, Lavie O, Assaf W, Cohen N, Sagi-Dain L, Bardicef M, et al. Changes in the obstetrical emergency department profile during the COVID-19 pandemic. The Journal of Maternal-Fetal & Neonatal Medicine. 2022;**35**(21):4116-4122

[19] Devakumar D, Shannon G, Bhopal SS, Abubakar I. Racism and discrimination in COVID-19 responses. Lancet (London, England). 2020;**395**(10231):1194

[20] Islam MS, Sarkar T, Khan SH, Kamal AHM, Hasan SM, Kabir A, et al. COVID–19–related information and its impact on public health: A global social media analysis. The American Journal of Tropical Medicine and Hygiene (London, United Kingdom). 2020;**103**(4):1621

[21] Jamili S, Ebrahimipour H, Adel A, Badiee Aval S, Hoseini SJ, Vejdani M, et al. Experience of patients hospitalized with COVID-19: A qualitative study of a pandemic disease in Iran. Health Expectations. 2022;**25**(2):513-521

[22] Alipour F, Arshi M, Ahmadi S, LeBeau R, Shaabani A, Ostadhashemi L. Psychosocial challenges and concerns of COVID-19: A qualitative study in Iran. Health. Nov 2022;**26**(6):702-719

[23] Schmidt T, Cloete A, Davids A, Makola L, Zondi N, Jantjies M. Myths, misconceptions, othering and stigmatizing responses to Covid-19 in South Africa: A rapid qualitative assessment. PLoS One. 2020;**15**(12):e0244420

[24] Tedros WDGD. Retraction of WHO Guidance on Opioid Use. United Nations Office; 2020

[25] Freeman D, Waite F, Rosebrock L, Petit A, Causier C, East A, et al. Coronavirus conspiracy beliefs, mistrust, and compliance with government guidelines in England. Psychological Medicine. 2020;**52**(2):1-30. DOI: 10.1017/S0033291720001890

[26] Gisondi MA, Barber R, Faust JS, Raja A, et al. A deadly infodemic: Social media and the power of COVID-19 misinformation. Journal of Medical Internet Research. 2022;**24**(2):e35552

[27] O'Brien M, McNicholas F. The use of telepsychiatry during COVID-19 and beyond. Irish Journal of Psychological Medicine (Cape Town, South Africa). 2020;**37**(4):250-255

[28] Chersich MF, Gray G, Fairlie L, et al. COVID-19 in Africa: Care and protection for frontline healthcare workers. Globalization and Health. 2020;**16**:46

[29] Lüdecke D, Von Dem Knesebeck O. Protective behavior in the course of the COVID-19 outbreak—Survey results from Germany. Frontiers in Public Health. 2020;**8**:572561

[30] Hoernke K, Djellouli N, Andrews L, et al. Frontline healthcare workers' experiences with personal protective equipment during the COVID-19 pandemic in the UK: A rapid qualitative appraisal. BMJ Open. 2021;**11**(1):e046199

Section 4

Quality Measurement, Performance, and Accountability in Primary Care

Chapter 6

Measuring Performance Quality in Health Care: Relevance and Validity of the Frameworks

Brahim Zaadoud and Youness Chbab

Abstract

Healthcare is the cornerstone of building a strong and high-performing health system. Performance evaluation in healthcare has become a key feature of many health systems in high-income countries. This research identifies the main performance measurement tools for healthcare quality, analyzes them, and highlights both strengths and areas for improvement. A qualitative analysis method was used to synthesize and organize the results of full-text studies included in the review based on three keywords: healthcare quality, healthcare performance, and performance measurement in healthcare. Fifteen (15) conceptual frameworks for measuring healthcare performance were identified, divided into two categories: Personal Models and Organizational Models. The results indicate that the majority of conceptual frameworks rely on Donabedian's model, with its triad of structure, process, and outcome, and there is a correlation between these three components within the context of quality systems.

Keywords: healthcare, indicators, frameworks, quality of care, performance

1. Introduction

Healthcare encompasses a wide range of services focused on maintaining health, preventing illnesses, diagnosing and treating medical conditions, and providing rehabilitation. These services vary widely and include both primary care as well as more specialized medical interventions, covering aspects such as disease prevention, health promotion, and therapeutic treatment. The ultimate aim of healthcare is to enhance the well-being of individuals and communities, ensuring that everyone has access to safe, effective, and high-quality healthcare services.

Healthcare can be classified into several categories:

1. *Primary healthcare*: This refers to the first point of contact between individuals and the healthcare system [1, 2]. Primary care services typically involve prevention, treatment, and basic community care, such as regular checkups, immunizations, and care for minor illnesses.

2. *Secondary healthcare*: This level includes more specialized medical services, including surgery and hospital-based treatments.

3. *Tertiary healthcare*: This is highly specialized care, often provided in major hospitals, such as intensive care units or treatments for complex diseases.

4. *Preventive healthcare*: Focused on reducing future health risks through education, vaccinations, and early detection programs.

Healthcare services not only address illnesses; they are also essential for promoting the overall health of the population.

1.1 The health system

A health system includes the governance structures, economic policies, and workforce development necessary to provide coordinated and high-quality healthcare services [3]. At its core, the health system is built on principles such as fairness, equitable access to services, community empowerment, self-determination, and cooperation across various sectors [4].

The *World Health Organization (WHO)* advocates for health systems that prioritize comprehensive medical care, with an emphasis on improving accessibility, providing a full range of services, and ensuring that specialized care is well-integrated [5].

To assess the performance of health systems, a comprehensive and integrated approach is essential. This approach considers various factors that impact the efficiency, effectiveness, and overall quality of healthcare. Successful health system performance requires alignment across multiple organizational functions.

Key components of health systems performance [6]:

1. *Service delivery*: Ensures that healthcare services are safe, accessible, and of high quality, meeting the needs of the population. This includes both preventive and curative care that is centered around the patient's needs.

2. *Resource management*: Involves the efficient allocation and use of financial, human, and material resources, minimizing waste and maximizing impact.

3. *Governance and leadership*: Encompasses the policies, regulations, and strategic direction that guide the healthcare system, emphasizing transparency, accountability, and evidence-based decision-making.

4. *Information systems*: Facilitates the collection, analysis, and dissemination of health data to support planning and evaluation, ensuring that decisions are data-driven.

5. *Equity and access*: Focuses on ensuring that healthcare services are available to all members of society, irrespective of their economic status, geographic location, or cultural background.

1.2 Performance measurement in healthcare

The objective of performance measurement in healthcare is twofold: improving the quality of care and enhancing accountability. Performance metrics in healthcare often focus on aspects like service delivery and the technical quality of medical procedures [7].

Publicly available performance data serves as a tool to promote transparency and accountability, enabling patients to select healthcare providers based on their performance and encouraging continuous improvement in areas where service quality may be lacking [8].

Because it is challenging to directly measure healthcare quality, performance is often assessed using multiple dimensions, including access to services, clinical and technical efficiency, equity in service delivery, and economic efficiency [9].

1.2.1 Conceptual frameworks for performance measurement

Various conceptual frameworks highlight that improving healthcare quality requires integrated strategies. These strategies often include patient assessments, evaluating health system operations, and focusing on key areas like safety, patient satisfaction, and overall healthcare effectiveness. Performance evaluation in health systems remains a critical issue globally, despite numerous efforts by governments, organizations, and healthcare providers to develop consistent measurement models [10]. Yet, there remains a lack of standardized frameworks, especially regarding the indicators and methods used for evaluation [11].

Over the years, several models have been developed to measure the quality of healthcare services [12]. These frameworks vary in terms of underlying principles and processes but share similar overall goals of improving healthcare standards [13, 14].

Performance measurement is considered an essential tool for driving continuous improvement in health systems. To be successful, the emphasis should be placed on patient-centered outcomes, strengthening the connection between quality measurement and accreditation systems, and advancing frameworks that help integrate existing models into practice. As noted by experts like Calva and McLean, while there is no conclusive proof that performance outcomes always lead to quality improvements, insights from other sectors suggest that performance measurement is vital for fostering change and innovation [15]. The role of quality measurement and accreditation systems will continue to grow in importance as healthcare systems evolve [16].

To ensure the consistent delivery of high-quality healthcare, it is critical to assess not only processes and outcomes but also patient experiences and the organizational frameworks that support care delivery. Shifting the focus from purely process measurement to outcomes that directly impact patients' lives is key to improving healthcare quality [17].

The goal of performance measurement in healthcare is to (a) achieve continuous improvement by identifying opportunities for improvement and tracking progress against organizational goals; (b) compare performance by benchmarking against internal and external standards; and (3) achieve desired results, including assessing the extent to which healthcare services meet their intended goals and focusing on evidence-based outcomes or processes [18].

2. Methods

2.1 Research objective

The objective of this study is to conduct a systematic review of the literature on frameworks and models for measurement in healthcare in order to identify conceptual frameworks for performance measurement in healthcare and strategies for improving them.

2.2 Search strategy

2.2.1 Study type

A qualitative analysis method was employed to synthesize and organize the results of full-text studies included in the review, based on three keywords: quality in healthcare, performance in healthcare, and performance measurement in healthcare. The research relied on databases such as MEDLINE, Google Scholar, Cochrane, and reference lists of studies to identify academic articles meeting the research criteria. The scope of the review was defined using a conceptual framework aimed at capturing factors relevant to performance evaluation in healthcare. Performance measurement and evaluation terms were combined using free text and guided terms. Only articles published in English and focusing on healthcare or community care were considered, while studies that did not address tools and mechanisms for measurement in healthcare were excluded. The review followed the steps outlined by Grant and Booth [19] in scientific research and adhered to PRISMA guidelines [20] for tracking published studies and descriptive analyses.

2.2.2 Qualitative data analysis

Thematic analysis was used, which consists of six steps: (1) *Data familiarization*: Reviewing and understanding the data; (2) *Coding*: Producing health-related codes for the data; (3) *Theme identification*: Identifying recurring themes; (4) *Reviewing themes*: Reviewing and refining the identified themes; (5) *Defining themes*: Clearly defining and describing the themes; (6) *Report preparation*: Structuring the findings into an organized report.

Articles were coded thematically to identify responses aligned with the selection criteria. Extracted data included theoretical foundations, measured constructs, and methods of development and evaluation of measurement properties.

2.2.3 Analysis stages

The selected studies were analyzed and categorized using the developed theoretical framework. Four stages were followed for data analysis: (1) collecting and categorizing information based on defined criteria; (2) analyzing obtained results; (3) creating comparative tables for existing conceptual frameworks; and (4) drawing conclusions and assessing performance for measurement frameworks.

3. Results

3.1 Literature base

The database search yielded 1245 articles, and 14 other items were identified by other sources, of which 562 were excluded due to duplicates and selection criteria. Six hundred and ninety-seven articles were screened by abstracts and titles. Four hundred and forty-seven articles were removed after review of abstracts and titles for relevance were further excluded; 140 articles were removed after scrutiny based on the inclusion criteria, leaving 37 articles for inclusion in the review. The literature search chart is shown in **Figure 1.**

This research highlights the significant expectations associated with the development of conceptual frameworks aimed at improving healthcare quality. Numerous established frameworks have been identified, many of which adapt or build upon existing models. These frameworks vary in terms of their structure, objectives, and the contexts in which they are applied. The findings underscore the lack of consensus regarding a single, universally accepted framework for enhancing healthcare quality, pointing to the ongoing need for efforts to create a unified global standard for measuring and improving healthcare performance. However, the diverse range of frameworks available offers researchers and healthcare managers a variety of tools and approaches, which can be advantageous in the quest for continuous quality improvement in healthcare systems [21].

This study reviews several extensive conceptual frameworks, drawing from both theoretical and applied evidence. It also evaluates the organization of healthcare systems and identifies specific areas where frameworks can be used for performance assessment, from practical, operational levels to broader systemic contexts.

Additionally, the review process involved tracking studies in the field of healthcare quality measurement and improvement. As a result, *fifteen conceptual frameworks* for measuring healthcare performance were identified. These were categorized into two groups: *Personal models* and *organizational models*.

Personal models include frameworks such as (1) the Donabedian model, (2) the Shortell model, (3) the Campbell model, (4) the Starfield model, (5) the Kringos model, (6) the Sicotte et al. model, (7) the EGIPSS model, and (8) the Kurk model.

Organizational models include frameworks such as (1) the WHO model, (2) the IOM model, (3) the Agency for Healthcare Research and Quality (AHRQ) model, (4) the Canadian model, (5) the Organization for Economic Co-operation Development (OECD) Member Countries model, (6) the Institute for Healthcare Improvement (IHI) model, and (7) the Australian model (see **Table 1**).

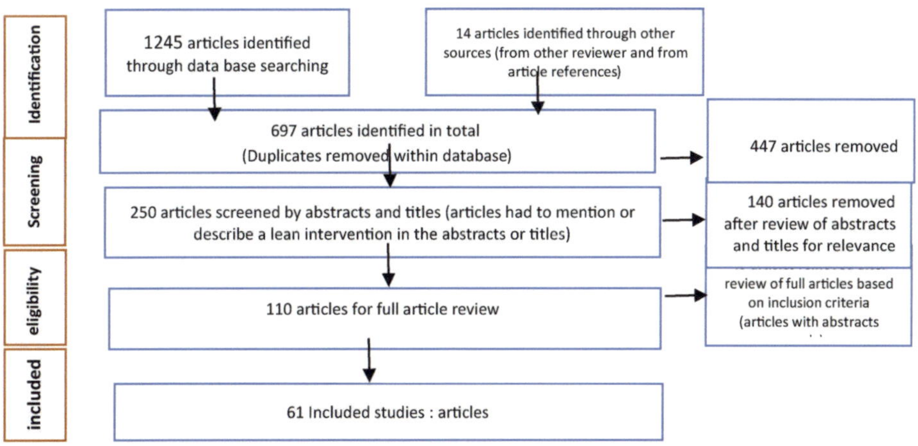

Figure 1.
Systematic review process.

The frameworks were diverse and categorized based on their structural composition, objectives, and contextual applications. A comprehensive comparison of these models can be seen in **Table 2**.

3.2 Individual models of conceptual frameworks for measuring performance in healthcare

3.2.1 Donabedian model (Donabedian A.)

In 1966, Donabedian pioneered the assessment of healthcare quality. His work led to the creation of the Donabedian model, which categorizes healthcare quality into three key components: structure, process, and outcome. The model considers both technical aspects of quality, such as efficiency and effectiveness, as well as functional aspects, including patient satisfaction. It is organized around four levels of evaluation: (1) the quality of care delivered by healthcare professionals; (2) the quality of the infrastructure used for patient care; (3) the benefits received by patients and their families; and (4) the quality of service delivery, focusing on access, continuity, and coordination of care.

3.2.2 Shortell et al. model

The Shortell model evaluates healthcare quality through four dimensions: strategic, cultural, technical, and structural [24]. The model highlights the importance of leadership, collaboration, and ongoing adaptation in driving performance improvements. It supports frameworks like the "patient-centered medical home" (PCMH) and the "accountable care organization" (ACO) [37]. Harrison et al. synthesized key

Framework	Authors	Years	Sources
Donabedian model	Donabedian Donabedian	1988 2005	The Quality of Care: How Can It Be Assessed? [22] Evaluating the Quality of Medical Care [23]
Shortell et al. model	Shortell et al.	2001	Assessing the impact of continuous quality improvement on clinical practice: what it will take to accelerate progress [24]
Campbell et al. model	Campbell et al. Campbell et al.	1999 2000	A developmental performance framework for primary care [25] Defining quality of care [26]
Starfield model	Starfield et al. Starfield et al.	2005 2008	Contribution of Primary Care to Health Systems and Health [27] Redesigning Primary Care [28]
Kringos et al. model	Kringos et al.	2010, a 2012	The European primary care monitor: structure, process and outcome indicators (2010) The strength of primary care in Europe [29]
Sicotte et al. model	Sicotte et al.	1998	A Conceptual Framework for the Analysis of Health Care Organizations' Performance (1998)
EGIPSS model	Champagne et al.	2005	A global evaluation framework for the performance of health service systems.
Kruk et al. model	Kruk et al.	2008	Assessing health system performance in developing countries: A review of the literature (2008)

Framework	Authors	Years	Sources
World Health Organization	World Health Organization	2000	The World Health Report 2000, Health Systems – Improving Performance, Geneva. (2000)
Institute of Medicine (IOM) model	Institute of Medicine	2001 2006	Crossing the Quality Chasm: A New Health System for the Twenty-First Century, Committee on Quality Health Care in America. Washington, DC: National Academy Press [30] Performance Measurement: Accelerating Improvement. Performance Measurement: Accelerating Improvement [31]
Agency for Healthcare Research and Quality (AHRQ) model	Agency for Healthcare Research and Quality	2016	Comparative Health System Performance Initiative: Compendium of U.S. Health Systems [32]
The Canadian model	Canadian Institute for Health Information Committee for the Ontario Primary Care Performance Measurement Initiative	2014 2017	A Primary Care Performance Measurement Framework for Ontario: Report of the Steering Committee for the Ontario Primary Care Performance Measurement Initiative: Phase One. Toronto: Queen's Printer for Ontario; [33]. Establishing a Primary Care Performance Measurement Framework for Ontario [34]
Organization for Economic Co-operation Development (OECD) model	Arah et al.	2006	A conceptual framework for the OECD Health Care Quality Indicators Project (2006)
Institute for Healthcare Improvement (IHI) model	Martin et al. Berwick et al.	2007 2008	Whole System Measures | IHI - Institute for Healthcare Improvement (2007) The Triple Aim: Care, Health, And Cost (2008)
The Australian National Health Performance model	Sibthorpe et al. The Australian National Health Performance	2007 2009	A Conceptual Framework for Performance Assessment in Primary Health Care [35] The National Health Performance Framework [36]

Table 1.
Sources of the conceptual model of performance measurement in primary health care.

elements from several influential frameworks, such as the Consolidated Framework for Implementation Research and the Socio-Ecological Framework, to address issues of patient orientation, care accountability, and population health management [38]. The model encompasses four levels of transformation: (1) individual patient responsibility; (2) teamwork and collaboration; (3) support for accountable care organizations; and (4) the environment in which care occurs [39].

3.2.3 Campbell et al. model

The Campbell model, building upon the Donabedian model, evaluates healthcare quality through two primary dimensions: access and effectiveness [26]. Effectiveness, in this context, includes both clinical outcomes and the personal relationships

Framework name	Angle analysis	Performance criteria	Evaluation of the performance	Results	Performance measurement matrices
Donabedian	Overall performance	Structures, processes, and outcomes as criteria for care quality.	Indicators of consistency, relevance, objectivity, specialization, and variance.	Considering the three performance levels: individual, organizational, and collective.	Balance between results and processes.
Shortell et al.	"Patient-centered care" and "Accountable care organization."	Four-dimensional framework: strategic, cultural, technical, and structural.	Focus on enablers and barriers within the four dimensions.	Providing integrated healthcare.	Four levels: patient, care team, organization, and the political and economic environment.
Campbell et al.	Two main dimensions: accessibility and effectiveness.	Structure, process, and outcome.	Differentiating quality from the perspective of individuals and populations.	Performance indicators.	Eight dimensions of performance.
Starfield	Organizational performance.	Delivery of primary care services.	Indicators to "measure" quality using a reliable and objective measurement system.	Elements such as human resources, facilities, and service organization.	Identifying the structural elements of health services like accessibility and continuity of service.
Kringos et al.	Measuring and comparing dimensions of primary care across countries.	Structure, process, and outcome.	Dimensions of primary care and their impact on outcomes.	Developing measurable health equity indicators oriented to primary care.	Three dimensions: governance, economic conditions, and workforce development. Four dimensions defining primary care processes: access, continuity, coordination, and comprehensiveness. Primary care system outcomes include three dimensions: care quality, efficiency, and health equity.
Sicotte et al.	Organizational performance.	Alignment of four organizational functions: 1. Coordination, 2. Integration, 3. Control, 4. Adaptation.	Specific performance criteria for each function and their coordination.	Measuring success indicators for each of the four organizational functions.	Network for reading organizational performance.

Framework name	Angle analysis	Performance criteria	Evaluation of the performance	Results	Performance measurement matrices
EGIPSS Model	Global and integrated evaluation of health systems performance.	A multidimensional model influenced by the efficiency and effectiveness of activities.	These indicators are related to access to services, continuity, comprehensiveness, and productivity.	Efficiency, effectiveness, responsiveness, productivity, quality, access, and equity, and relies on organizational performance. Each indicator reflects clinical and organizational practices, resource availability, and the specific environment.	Five elements for evaluating healthcare services performance: 1. the evaluation objective; 2. performance perception; 3. evaluation objectives and target audience; 4. preferred values; and 5. operational feasibility.
Kruk et al.	Performance analysis of primary healthcare structures.	Four dimensions: effectiveness, efficiency, equity, and satisfaction.	Performance analysis from the perspective of caregivers and beneficiaries.	Comparing measured performance evaluations.	Identifying causes and risks, and evaluating intervention strategies and techniques.
World Health Organization	Four key functions: financing, service delivery, resource generation, and system management.	Performance variations based on healthcare system organization.	Three main goals: improving health, enhancing responsiveness, and ensuring financial equity.	WHO model focuses on efficiency and "outcomes achieved relative to resources."	Six interconnected dimensions: clinical effectiveness, safety, patient-centeredness, governance, staff orientation, and efficiency.
Institute of Medicine (IOM)	Improving care experience, population health, and cost reduction.	Partnership with individuals and families, primary care redesign, and population health management.	Comparison for performance measurement.	Reducing service delivery errors.	Six dimensions: safety, effectiveness, patient-centeredness, timeliness, efficiency, and equity.
Agency for Healthcare Research and Quality (AHRQ)	Three main objectives for measuring diagnostic safety: 1. Determine diagnostic error rates. 2. Identify causes and risks of errors. 3. Assess the effectiveness of strategies and interventions.	Comprehensive health system: quality indicators for primary care prevention and safety.	Specifications of indicators for providers and physicians: quality prevention indicators linked to primary care.	Learning from participants and identifying future research trends.	Three axes: 1. Learning from ideas and experiences shared by participants. 2. Studying issues related to definitions, physicians' and patients' perspectives, data usage and measurement, the role of health IT, and the impact of organizational factors on diagnosis. 3. Identifying potential future research directions.

Framework name	Angle analysis	Performance criteria	Evaluation of the performance	Results	Performance measurement matrices
The Canadian Model	Health, financial, material, and human resources.	Core dimensions: quality, accessibility, and expenditure.	Quality core dimensions: accessibility, efficiency, and equity.	Comprehensive evaluation of the impact of organizational models on primary care outcomes, including acceptability, accessibility, appropriateness, continuity, effectiveness, efficiency, equity, patient focus, and safety.	Four pillars: 1. Providing faster access to appropriate care. 2. Improving home and community care through community integration. 3. Providing information for making the right health decisions. 4. Ensuring the sustainability of the universal healthcare system for future generations.
Organization for Economic Co-operation and Development (OECD)	Developing a set of indicators to compare healthcare quality among OECD member countries.	Two main components: 1. Delivery of healthcare services. 2. Technical quality of clinical care.	Improving quality and enhancing accountability.	Quality indicators include effectiveness, efficiency, safety, and quality. Indicators must provide: 1. A quality goal. 2. A concept for measurement. 3. A concept for evaluation.	Multiple quality domains: acceptability, continuity, efficiency, and sustainability.
Institute for Healthcare Improvement (IHI)	"Triple Aim": Improving the individual care experience, improving population health, and reducing individual healthcare costs in communities.	Developing whole system measures, a balanced set of system-level measures, a useful conceptual framework for organizing healthcare quality measures, a specific set of quality indicators contributing to the measures set of a healthcare organization, a balanced scorecard, or a strategic performance measures dashboard.	Developing and using a balanced system measure aligned with the Triple Aim.	Focus on five components: 1. Individuals and families; 2. Redesigning primary care services and structures; 3. Population health management; 4. Cost control platform; 5. System integration and implementation.	A set of system-level measures includes methods for tracking care experience in outpatient settings, including patient engagement, continuity, and preventive clinical practices.

Framework name	Angle analysis	Performance criteria	Evaluation of the performance	Results	Performance measurement matrices
The Australian National Health Performance	Three levels: 1. Health status and outcomes. 2. Health determinants. 3. Health system performance.	Linking results with processes in the context of a specific program.	It contains four levels: 1. Governance 2. Organizational structures and processes 3. Care processes 4. Intermediate outcomes.	Includes two levels focusing on organizational structures and processes, with one for divisions and another for general practices supported.	Covers "Health Status and Outcomes," "Health Determinants," and "Health System Performance." Includes two levels focusing on "Organizational Structures and Processes," one for departments and another for general practices supported.

Table 2.
Comparison of performance measurement models of quality of care around the world according to performance criteria.

between patients and providers [35]. The model identifies four key outcomes: health status, patient evaluation, cost of service delivery, and equity. Additionally, it incorporates eight performance dimensions that include specific and non-specific skills, communication abilities (both written and oral), effort estimation, self-discipline, teamwork, supervision, and management.

3.2.4 Starfield model

The Starfield model focuses on four core principles of primary care: (1) *first-contact access*, which involves delivering timely care while minimizing barriers; (2) *continuity*, which emphasizes the ongoing relationship between patients and providers; (3) *comprehensiveness*, offering a wide range of services that address prevention, diagnosis, treatment, and rehabilitation; and (4) *coordination*, ensuring that healthcare services are integrated across different levels of care [5]. Derived features include accessibility, service range, and utilization. The model is grounded in core values such as *equity*, ensuring universal access to healthcare, *efficiency*, optimizing resource use, and *effectiveness*, ensuring care meets desired outcomes [40]. The Starfield model argues that a strong primary care foundation leads to better overall public health outcomes, reduced mortality, and diminished health disparities.

3.2.5 Kringos et al. model

Kringos' framework defines the healthcare system as a multifaceted entity contributing to health outcomes through multiple dimensions. These include governance, economic conditions, workforce development, access to care, continuity, coordination, comprehensiveness, quality, effectiveness, and health equity [3]. The model aims to explore the interactions between these dimensions to assess how each contributes to health system performance. These dimensions ensure that healthcare is delivered efficiently and effectively, providing equitable access across all societal segments, including vulnerable populations.

3.2.6 Sicotte et al. model

This model focuses on four critical functions within healthcare organizations (HCOs): coordination, integration, control, and adaptation. These functions interact dynamically, resulting in a balance that affects organizational performance. The model's strength lies in its ability to combine traditional performance models, offering a unified framework that captures multiple performance dimensions. For example, *coordination* ensures that resources and activities are efficiently aligned across different levels of care, while *integration* promotes collaboration across healthcare sectors. *Control* ensures the monitoring and regulation of performance through quality assurance and accountability mechanisms, while *adaptation* involves the organization's ability to respond to internal and external changes, fostering long-term sustainability [41].

3.2.7 EGIPSS model

The Global and Integrated Evaluation of Health Systems Performance (EGIPSS) model is a comprehensive framework for assessing healthcare performance. It is based on principles such as efficiency, effectiveness, responsiveness, quality, access, and equity. The model emphasizes the need to align organizational functions—such as service delivery, resource management, and governance—through clear objectives and integrated processes. This alignment ensures that all parts of the healthcare system work cohesively to enhance outcomes. Performance is monitored through data-driven feedback, and flexibility is encouraged to adapt to emerging challenges like demographic shifts and health crises [42]. The model ultimately aims to enhance the system's ability to respond to patient and community needs, ensuring equity and resilience in dynamic healthcare environments.

3.2.8 Kruk et al. model

Kruk et al.'s model provides a framework for evaluating primary healthcare systems based on four essential dimensions: *effectiveness*, *efficiency*, *equity*, and *satisfaction*. The model emphasizes the importance of using health information systems to assess performance and enhance quality across these dimensions [43]. By focusing on these four areas, the model aims to ensure that primary healthcare systems are meeting their health goals, utilizing resources efficiently, ensuring fair access for all populations, and achieving high levels of satisfaction from both healthcare providers and recipients [44]. This model emphasizes the need for integrated care processes that not only consider final outcomes but also the quality of care delivery.

3.3 Models of organizations

3.3.1 World Health Organization (WHO) model

The *World Health Report 2000* [45] identified four key functions in the health system: financing, service delivery, resource generation, and the administrative system, which includes oversight of both public and private sectors. The report also outlined three overarching goals for the health system: promoting good health for populations, ensuring responsiveness to public needs, and ensuring equitable financing mechanisms [10]. These goals aim to improve health outcomes, enhance system responsiveness to the expectations of populations, and promote financial fairness. The responsiveness of the system is built on two elements: (1) respect for individuals and (2) a client-centered approach.

Variations in performance are attributed to how the system organizes its core functions: governance, financing, service delivery, and resource generation. The WHO model emphasizes *efficiency*, which refers to the measurable outcomes of the health system's performance. With growing concerns about safety in care, this model has become integral to discussions around healthcare reforms [46]. The WHO framework is grounded in six interconnected dimensions: clinical effectiveness, safety, patient-centered care, responsive governance, staff orientation, and overall efficiency.

3.3.2 American Institute of Medicine (IOM) model

The *Institute of Medicine (IOM)* model has long been a foundational framework for healthcare reform planning and assessing healthcare quality in the U.S. This model focuses on three primary goals: improving the personal care experience, enhancing population health, and reducing healthcare costs [47]. Five integrated components guide the model: partnerships with individuals and families, redesigning healthcare, population health management, financial management, and system integration.

The IOM's emphasis on improving quality centers around six key dimensions: safety, effectiveness, patient-centeredness, timeliness, efficiency, and equity [30]. The framework promotes ongoing reevaluation and adjustment of strategies, policies, and programs to ensure that the system evolves to meet these goals effectively [48].

3.3.3 Agency for Healthcare Research and Quality (AHRQ) model

The *AHRQ model* focuses on measuring healthcare quality by identifying diagnostic error rates, determining the root causes of errors, and evaluating the effectiveness of interventions. To meet these objectives, the model relies on insights from stakeholders, including physicians and patients, utilizing data, measurement systems, health IT, and organizational factors [49]. It also highlights future research directions to further improve healthcare delivery and error management.

3.3.4 Canadian model

The Canadian healthcare system, as highlighted by *Watson et al.*, is supported by substantial government contributions in terms of financial, material, and human resources [50]. The model emphasizes the importance of timely and accessible care, with a particular focus on primary care, team-based interdisciplinary approaches, chronic disease management, and healthcare sustainability.

In Canada, the key objectives of the healthcare model include ensuring (1) timely access to care, (2) efficient home and community-based services, (3) accurate health information for informed decision-making, and (4) the long-term sustainability of the healthcare system [51]. The model also evaluates primary care outcomes through metrics such as access, suitability, continuity, effectiveness, efficiency, equity, patient focus, and safety.

3.3.5 Organization for Economic Co-operation and Development (OECD) member countries model

The *OECD model* aims to compare healthcare quality across its member countries using a set of standardized indicators. The OECD health quality indicators project underscores the complexity of healthcare and the need for a balanced framework that integrates key concepts and performance dimensions. The model is divided into two components: healthcare service delivery and clinical care technical quality [52]. The objectives of measuring healthcare quality include improving overall performance and enhancing accountability.

Several key quality areas are identified by Arah and colleagues, such as access to services, care environment, expenditures, governance, efficiency, continuity, patient-centered care, safety, and timeliness. These indicators provide a comprehensive overview of healthcare performance, allowing for comparison across countries and systems [53].

3.3.6 Institute for Healthcare Improvement (IHI) model

The *IHI model* focuses on improving healthcare quality by implementing strategies that enhance the efficiency and effectiveness of services. The IHI developed a comprehensive system-level approach that includes a set of balanced measures to monitor quality of care across various healthcare organizations [54]. This system is closely aligned with the "Triple Aim" framework, which seeks to improve the patient experience, improve population health, and reduce healthcare costs [47]. The model includes essential components such as (1) patient-centered care, (2) collaboration among healthcare teams, (3) performance measurement through data analysis, (4) continuous learning, and (5) sustainable improvements in health outcomes. The goal is to reduce medical errors and enhance health outcomes through teamwork and ongoing improvements in healthcare delivery. The IHI's approach provides a holistic view of care that encompasses patient participation, continuity, and preventive practices.

3.3.7 Australian national healthcare model

The *Australian national healthcare model* was developed to address two primary concerns: (1) effective resource allocation and (2) improving the quality of healthcare. The *Australian Institute of Health and Welfare (AIHW)* established guiding principles for performance indicators, which emphasize comprehensive and equitable access to healthcare services, a focus on prevention, and ensuring high-quality care in all settings. This model incorporates three levels of healthcare performance: (1) health status and outcomes, (2) health determinants, and (3) health system performance [55]. These outcomes are linked to various programmatic processes, with four primary levels of focus: governance, organizational structures and processes, care processes, and intermediate outcomes. Key dimensions in the Australian model include quality, equity, efficiency, effectiveness, access, safety, and continuity of care.

4. Discussion

The *2008 World Health Organization (WHO)* report, titled *"Primary Health Care – Now More Than Ever,"* underscored the importance of advancing knowledge production within healthcare [56]. Measuring and evaluating healthcare quality is critical for several reasons: (1) to understand the mechanisms, benefits, and risks associated with healthcare systems; (2) to assess the impact and relevance of interventions; and (3) to evaluate their role in reducing health inequalities, particularly in terms of structure, processes, and outcomes [28].

Experts in the field disagree on a unified definition of healthcare quality. According to *Beyan and Baykal*, assessing healthcare quality requires first defining what "quality" means in the context of health services [57]. *Starfield* [5] noted that defining and managing "good healthcare" remains ambiguous and is continually evolving. This ambiguity stems from several factors: each healthcare delivery system has unique features, different metrics serve distinct improvement goals, and healthcare systems are complex, multifaceted organizations whose processes cannot be reduced to a single, universally applicable performance metric [5]. Consequently, evaluations and comparisons must reflect this inherent complexity. Additionally, performance measurement models are highly context-dependent and must be tailored to the specific needs of each healthcare system.

A study by *Jackson et al.* indicated that although quality measurement frameworks share common goals—such as improving care coordination and enhancing service access—their definitions and methods of implementation differ substantially

[58]. *Lamarche et al.* concluded that organizational models significantly influence healthcare outcomes, with variations in performance largely linked to factors like organizational vision and the broader environmental context [59]. *Sutton and McLean* emphasized that aspects such as team size and financial incentives can independently impact care quality [60].

Kringos et al. [3] argued that healthcare systems contribute to overall system performance and population health through their structural and procedural dimensions. According to *Kunkel et al.* [61], systems that score highly in both structure and process evaluations also tend to excel in implementation, especially when there is robust collaboration between managers and frontline staff. Effective healthcare is often associated with positive outcomes and lower costs.

Beyan and Baykal [57] reinforced that performance measurement is key to improving healthcare systems, but noted that no universally accepted performance measurement framework currently exists. *Klassen et al.* [62] highlighted that the most significant takeaway from the array of healthcare performance frameworks is the identification of common quality principles.

To effectively measure performance, healthcare goals must be clearly defined to improve patient safety and care quality. Evaluations should address the core dimensions of healthcare within the context of the specific system. Therefore, refining performance objectives for healthcare organizations and assessing whether sound management practices can improve performance is essential.

Porter [17] emphasized that the ultimate goal of outcome measurement is to identify opportunities for learning, as no healthcare practice excels in all areas. *Kadri and Peyton* [63] identified four essential pillars for effective performance measurement models: (1) improving system integration and access, (2) modernizing individual and community care, (3) enhancing population health and well-being, and (4) ensuring system sustainability and quality.

Ramani et al. [64] suggested that a sustainable performance measurement framework should include a focus on sustainability, the development of clear goals, the application of performance metrics, ongoing refinement of the framework, and the continuous application of feedback.

Most performance measurement frameworks highlight the importance of developing quality indicators and routine care processes as crucial steps in improving healthcare quality. *Braithwaite et al.* [65] noted that performance indicators have become valuable tools for measuring healthcare quality and promoting continuous improvement in healthcare systems.

However, *Kadri and Peyton* [63] argued that these frameworks hold little value unless they generate actionable feedback and sufficient evidence for corrective action. *Fekri et al.* [66] reported that many healthcare performance frameworks are poorly integrated with routine information systems and national health priorities. Additionally, managing organizations solely based on performance objectives can lead to unintended, dysfunctional consequences.

While the measurement of healthcare dimensions remains a challenging and often limited process, progress is being made. These frameworks play a vital role in evaluating and enhancing healthcare performance. They emphasize the importance of quality across structure, process, and outcome, while also focusing on leadership, innovation, access, equity, and coordination among providers. Performance measurement systems are essential tools for implementing these frameworks and fostering continuous improvement in healthcare.

5. Limitations

Several challenges were encountered in this study: the ambiguous nature of the topic made it difficult to identify and review relevant literature; developing a search strategy that adequately balanced recall and precision was challenging; important information may have been overlooked; the use of non-validated tools for performance evaluation presents a significant limitation; and there was some subjectivity in determining which frameworks were eligible for inclusion in the review. Furthermore, establishing causal links between healthcare dimensions and outcomes was challenging, as noted by *Kringos et al.* [3].

6. Conclusion

This study highlights the diverse processes and methodologies used to develop performance measurement frameworks in healthcare. Performance measurement is widely considered a key tool for achieving continuous improvement in health systems. The findings suggest that most conceptual frameworks are grounded in *Donabedian's* model, which includes the triad of structure, process, and outcome. These components are interdependent within the context of quality systems.

Success depends on measuring outcomes that directly impact patient health, strengthening the integration between quality measurement systems and accreditation, and developing conceptual frameworks that enhance the practical application of existing models. Most performance measurement models derive their core concepts from foundational frameworks introduced by scholars such as *Donabedian*, *Starfield*, *Kunkel*, *Kringos*, and *Shortell*, as well as from broader concepts like systems thinking and key dimensions such as capacity, performance, health policies, and performance indicators for health groups. These frameworks emphasize interconnected dimensions, including cultural, technical, and structural strategies, organizational performance, and coordinated exchanges among healthcare providers.

7. Future research in quality management systems

Future research should focus on:

- Establishing causal links between management strategies and quality outcomes, particularly in relation to patient safety.

- Moving beyond linear models of healthcare quality measurement to include multiple perspectives and levels, given the complexity of healthcare systems.

- Verifying the implementation of quality systems and linking these processes to historical performance data of departments within quality management frameworks.

- Assessing the feasibility of achieving specific quality objectives, as some goals may be more attainable than others.

8. Key messages

- Most primary care is provided in general practice.
- Research in this area does not provide a complete picture of the quality of primary care in terms of methodological rigor and comprehensiveness.
- Most of the studies that examined the quality of care did not achieve acceptable standards of practice.
- Stakeholders should strive to improve the quality of primary health care.

Author details

Brahim Zaadoud[1*] and Youness Chbab[2]

1 Faculty of Medicine and Pharmacy, Clinical Neurosciences Laboratory, University of Fez, Ministry of Health, Morocco

2 Institute of Specialized Health Professionals, University of My Slimane Bni Mellal, Morocco

*Address all correspondence to: zaadoud@gmail.com

References

[1] Lawn JE, Rohde J, Rifkin S, Were M, Paul VK, Chopra M. Alma-Ata 30 years on: Revolutionary, relevant, and time to revitalise. Lancet (London, England). 2008;**372**(9642):917-927. DOI: 10.1016/S0140-6736(08)61402-6

[2] Shi L et al. Clinical quality performance in U.S. health centers. Health Services Research. 2012;**47**(6):2225-2249. DOI: 10.1111/j.1475-6773.2012.01418.x

[3] Kringos DS, Boerma WG, Hutchinson A, van der Zee J, Groenewegen PP. The breadth of primary care: A systematic literature review of its core dimensions. BMC Health Services Research. 2010a;**10**(1):Art. no 1. DOI: 10.1186/1472-6963-10-65

[4] Keleher H. Why primary health care offers a more comprehensive approach to tackling health inequities than primary care. Australian Journal of Primary Health. 2001;7(2):57-61. DOI: 10.1071/py01035

[5] Starfield B. Primary care and equity in health: The importance to effectiveness and equity of responsiveness to peoples' needs. Humanity and Society. 2009;**33**(1-2):56-73. DOI: 10.1177/016059760903300105

[6] Adam T, de Savigny D. Systems thinking for strengthening health systems in LMICs: Need for a paradigm shift. Health Policy and Planning. 2012;**27**(suppl_4):iv1-iv3. DOI: 10.1093/heapol/czs084

[7] Haggerty J et al. Operational definitions of attributes of primary health care: Consensus among Canadian experts. Annals of Family Medicine. 2007;**5**(4):336-344. DOI: 10.1370/afm.682

[8] Marshall M et al. OECD health care quality indicator project. The expert panel on primary care prevention and health promotion. International Journal for Quality in Health Care. 2006;**18**(suppl_1):21-25. DOI: 10.1093/intqhc/mzl021

[9] Fung CH, Lim Y-W, Mattke S, Damberg C, Shekelle PG. Systematic review: The evidence that publishing patient care performance data improves quality of care. Annals of Internal Medicinc. 2008. [En ligne]. Disponible sur: https://www.acpjournals.org/doi/10.7326/0003-4819-148-2-200801150-00006 [Consulté le: janvier 13, 2025]

[10] Murray CJL, Evans DB, Evans DB, O. mondiale de la santé. Health Systems Performance Assessment: Debates, Methods and Empiricism. World Health Organization; 2003

[11] Kazandjian VA, Matthes N, Wicker KG. Are Performance Indicators Generic? The International Experience of the Quality Indicator Project®. 2003. [En ligne]. Disponible sur: https://onlinelibrary.wiley.com/doi/10.1046/j.1365-2753.2003.00374.x [Consulté le: janvier 13, 2025]

[12] Lanier DC, Roland M, Burstin H, Knottnerus JA. Doctor performance and public accountability. The Lancet. 2003;**362**(9393):1404-1408. DOI: 10.1016/S0140-6736(03)14638-7

[13] Groene O, Botje D, Suñol R, Lopez MA, Wagner C. A systematic review of instruments that assess the implementation of hospital quality management systems. International Journal for Quality in Health Care. 2013;**25**(5):525-541. DOI: 10.1093/intqhc/mzt058

[14] Ovretveit J. Leading improvement. Journal of Health Organization and Management. 2005;**19**(6):413-430. DOI: 10.1108/14777260510629661

[15] Galvin R, McGlynn EA. Using Performance Measurement to Drive Improvement: A Road...: Medical Care. LWW. [En ligne]. Disponible sur: https://journals.lww.com/lww-medicalcare/fulltext/2003/01001/using_performance_measurement_to_drive.6.aspx [Consulté le: janvier 13, 2025]

[16] Chuang S, Howley PP, Hancock S. Using clinical indicators to facilitate quality improvement via the accreditation process: An adaptive study into the control relationship. International Journal for Quality in Health Care. 2013;**25**(3):277-283. DOI: 10.1093/intqhc/mzt023

[17] Porter ME, Pabo EA, Lee TH. Redesigning primary care: A strategic vision to improve value by organizing around patients' needs. Health Affairs (Millwood). 2013;**32**(3):516-525. DOI: 10.1377/hlthaff.2012.0961

[18] Health Quality Ontario. Health Quality Ontario's Releases 2015 Measuring up Report|AFHTO. [En ligne]. Disponible sur: https://www.afhto.ca/news-events/news/health-quality-ontarios-releases-2015-measuring-report [Consulté le: janvier 20, 2025]

[19] Grant MJ, Booth A. A Typology of Reviews: An Analysis of 14 Review Types and Associated Methodologies. 2009. [En ligne]. Disponible sur: https://onlinelibrary.wiley.com/doi/10.1111/j.1471-1842.2009.00848.x [Consulté le: janvier 13, 2025]

[20] Moher D, Altman DG, Tetzlaff AL, Liberati A, Tetzlaff J. Preferred reporting items for systematic reviews and meta-analyses: The PRISMA statement. BMJ. 2009;**339**:b2535. DOI: 10.1136/bmj.b2535

[21] Langton JM et al. Primary care performance measurement and reporting at a regional level: Could a matrix approach provide actionable information for policy makers and clinicians? Healthcare Policy. 2016;**12**(2):33. [En ligne]. Disponible sur: https://pmc.ncbi.nlm.nih.gov/articles/PMC5221710/ [Consulté le: janvier 13, 2025]

[22] Donabedian A. The quality of care how can it be assessed? JAMA. 1988

[23] Donabedian A. Evaluating the quality of medical care. The Milbank Quarterly. 2005;**83**(4):691. DOI: 10.1111/j.1468-0009.2005.00397.x

[24] Shortell SM, Bennett CL, Byck GR. Assessing the Impact of Continuous Quality Improvement on Clinical Practice: What it Will Take to Accelerate Progress. 2001. [En ligne]. Disponible sur: https://onlinelibrary.wiley.com/doi/10.1111/1468-0009.00107 [Consulté le: janvier 13, 2025]

[25] Proctor S, Campbell J. A developmental performance framework for primary care. International Journal of Health Care Quality Assurance Incorporating Leadership in Health Services. 1999

[26] Campbell SM, Roland MO, Buetow SA. Defining quality of care. Social Science & Medicine. 2000;**51**(11):1611-1625. DOI: 10.1016/S0277-9536(00)00057-5

[27] Starfield B, Shi L, Macinko J. Contribution of Primary Care to Health Systems and Health. 2005. [En ligne]. Disponible sur: https://onlinelibrary.wiley.com/

doi/10.1111/j.1468-0009.2005.00409.x [Consulté le: juillet 19, 2025]

[28] Lee TH, Bodenheimer T, Goroll AH, Starfield B, Treadway K. Redesigning primary care. The New England Journal of Medicine. [En ligne]. Disponible sur: https://www.nejm.org/doi/full/10.1056/NEJMp0809050 [Consulté le: janvier 13, 2025]

[29] Kringos DS. The Strength of Primary Care in Europe = De sterkte van de eerste lijn in Europa. Utrecht: Nivel; 2012

[30] Institute of Medicine. Crossing the Quality Chasm: A New Health System for the 21st Century. Washington (DC): National Academies Press (US); 2001. [En ligne]. Disponible sur: http://www.ncbi.nlm.nih.gov/books/NBK222274/ [Consulté le: novembre 22, 2021]

[31] Institute of Medicine, Performance Measurement. Board on Health Care Services, Committee on Redesigning Health Insurance Performance Measures, Payment, and Performance Improvement Programs. 2006. [En ligne]. Disponible sur: https://books.google.com/books/about/Performance_Measurement.html?hl=fr&id=DTYZJwbCvTgC [Consulté le: juillet 19, 2025]

[32] Agency for Healthcare Research and Quality. Comparative Health System Performance Initiative: Compendium of U.S. Health Systems. [En ligne]. Disponible sur: http://www.ahrq.gov/chsp/data-resources/compendium/technical-documentation.html [Consulté le: septembre 4, 2020]

[33] Health Quality Ontario. A Primary Care Performance Measurement Framework for Ontario- Report of the Steering Committee for the Ontario Primary Care Performance Measurement Initiative: Phase One. 2014

[34] Haj-Ali W, Hutchison B. Establishing a primary care performance measurement framework for Ontario. Healthcare Policy. 2017;**12**(3):66-79. [En ligne]. Disponible sur: https://www.ncbi.nlm.nih.gov/pmc/articles/PMC5344364/ [Consulté le: septembre 14, 2020]

[35] Sibthorpe B, Gardner K. A conceptual framework for performance assessment in primary health care. Australian Journal of Primary Health. 2007;**13**(2):96-103. DOI: 10.1071/py07027

[36] Bennett CC. National Health and Hospitals Reform Commission 2009, A Healthier Future for all Australians – Final Report of the National Health and Hospitals Reform Commission, NHHRC, Canberra. [En ligne]. Disponible sur: https://www.researchgate.net/publication/26874703_National_Health_and_Hospitals_Reform_Commission_2009_A_Healthier_Future_for_All_Australians_-_Final_Report_of_the_National_Health_and_Hospitals_Reform_Commission_NHHRC_Canberra [Consulté le: juillet 19, 2025]

[37] Singer SJ, Burgers J, Friedberg M, Rosenthal MB, Leape L, Schneider E. Defining and measuring integrated patient care: Promoting the next frontier in health care delivery. Medical Care Research and Review. 2011;**68**(1):112-127. DOI: 10.1177/1077558710371485

[38] Harrison MI, Shortell SM. Multi-level analysis of the learning health system: Integrating contributions from research on organizations and implementation. Learning Health Systems. 2020:e10226. DOI: 10.1002/lrh2.10226

[39] Shortell SM, Gillies R, Wu F. United States innovations in healthcare delivery. Public Health Reviews. 2010;**32**(1):190-212. DOI: 10.1007/BF03391598

[40] Starfield B. Toward international primary care reform. CMAJ. 2009;**180**(11):1091-1092. DOI: 10.1503/cmaj.090542

[41] Sicotte C et al. A conceptual framework for the analysis of health care organizations' performance. Health Services Management Research. 1998;**11**(1):24-41. DOI: 10.1177/095148489801100106

[42] Champagne F, Contandriopoulos' A-P, Picot-Touché J, Beland F, Nguyen H. A Framework for Evaluating the Performance of Health Service Systems: The EGIPSS Model. 2005

[43] Barry AM. Évaluation de la performance des structures des soins de santé primaires du district sanitaire de Labé (Guinée). 2011. [En ligne]. Disponible sur: https://papyrus.bib.umontreal.ca/xmlui/handle/1866/5275 [Consulté le: septembre 27, 2020]

[44] Kruk ME, Freedman LP. Assessing health system performance in developing countries: A review of the literature. Health Policy. 2008;**85**(3):263-276. DOI: 10.1016/j.healthpol.2007.09.003

[45] WHO. Health Systems: Improving Performance. The World Health Report. World Health Organization; 2000. [En ligne]. Disponible sur: https://apps.who.int/iris/handle/10665/42281 [Consulté le: avril 5, 2021]

[46] Veillard J, Champagne F, Klazinga N, Kazandjian V, Arah OA, Guisset A-L. A performance assessment framework for hospitals: The WHO regional office for Europe PATH project. International Journal for Quality in Health Care. 2005;**17**(6):487-496. DOI: 10.1093/intqhc/mzi072

[47] Berwick DM, Nolan TW, Whittington J. The triple aim: Care, health, and cost. Health Affairs (Millwood). 2008;**27**(3):759-769. DOI: 10.1377/hlthaff.27.3.759

[48] Veillard J, Garcia-Armesto S, Kadandale S, Klazinga N, Leatherman S. International health system comparisons: From measurement challenge to management tool. In: Smith PC, Mossialos E, Papanicolas I, editors. Performance Measurement for Health System Improvement. Cambridge: Cambridge University Press; 2010. pp. 641-672. DOI: 10.1017/CBO9780511711800.023

[49] Henriksen K, Dymek C, Harrison MI, Brady PJ, Arnold SB. Challenges and opportunities from the Agency for Healthcare Research and Quality (AHRQ) research summit on improving diagnosis: A proceedings review. Diagnosis. 2017;**4**(2):57-66. DOI: 10.1515/dx-2017-0016

[50] Watson DE, Broemeling A-M, Wong ST. A results-based logic model for primary healthcare: A conceptual foundation for population-based information systems. Healthcare Policy. 2009;**5**(Spec No):33. [En ligne]. Disponible sur: https://pmc.ncbi.nlm.nih.gov/articles/PMC2906214/ [Consulté le: janvier 13, 2025]

[51] Mandate letter. Health and Long-Term Care. [En ligne]. Disponible sur: https://www.ontario.ca/page/september-2016-mandate-letter-health-and-long-term-care [Consulté le: septembre 12, 2020]

[52] OECD and W. H. Organization. Improving Healthcare Quality in Europe Characteristics, Effectiveness and Implementation of Different Strategies. OECD Publishing; 2019

[53] Arah OA, Westert GP, Hurst J, Klazinga NS. A conceptual framework for the OECD health care quality

indicators project. International Journal for Quality in Health Care. 2006;**18**(suppl_1):5-13. DOI: 10.1093/intqhc/mzl024

[54] Martin J, Spano A. From performance management to strategic local government leadership: Lessons from different cultural settings. Public Money & Management. 2015;**35**(4):303-310. DOI: 10.1080/09540962.2015.1047276

[55] Bennett V, McIntyre J. Australia's Health 2008; Health System Performance. Australian Institute of Health and Welfare. [En ligne]. Disponible sur: https://www.aihw.gov.au/reports/australias-health/australias-health-2008/contents/table-of-contents; [Consulté le: janvier 13, 2025]

[56] WHO. The World Health Report 2008. 2008. [En ligne]. Disponible sur: https://books.google.com/books/about/The_World_Health_Report_2008.html?hl=fr&id=q-EGxRjrIo4C [Consulté le: janvier 13, 2025]

[57] Beyan OD, Baykal N. A knowledge based search tool for performance measures in health care systems. Journal of Medical Systems. 2012;**36**(1):201-221. DOI: 10.1007/s10916-010-9459-2

[58] Jackson GL et al. The patient-centered medical home. Annals of Internal Medicine. 2013;**158**(3):169-178. DOI: 10.7326/0003-4819-158-3-201302050-00579

[59] Lamarche T. Le territoire entre politique de développement et attractivité. Études de Communication. Langages, Information, Médiations. 2003;**26**:Art No 26. DOI: 10.4000/edc.122

[60] Sutton M, McLean G. Determinants of primary medical care quality measured under the new UK contract: Cross sectional study. BMJ. 2006;**332**(7538):389-390. DOI: 10.1136/bmj.38742.554468.55

[61] Kunkel S, Rosenqvist U, Westerling R. Implementation strategies influence the structure, process and outcome of quality systems: An empirical study of hospital departments in Sweden. Quality & Safety in Health Care. 2009;**18**(1):49-54. DOI: 10.1136/qshc.2007.023978

[62] Klassen A, Miller A, Anderson N, Shen J, Schiariti V, O'Donnell M. Performance measurement and improvement frameworks in health, education and social services systems: A systematic review. International Journal for Quality in Health Care. 2010;**22**(1):44-69. DOI: 10.1093/intqhc/mzp057

[63] Kadri NE, Peyton L. A systematic literature review comparing primary and community health care indicators and measurement frameworks. Procedia Computer Science. 2017;**113**:384-391. DOI: 10.1016/j.procs.2017.08.353

[64] Ramani TL, Zietsman J, Gudmundsson H, Hall RP, Marsden G. Framework for sustainability assessment by transportation agencies. Transportation Research Record. 2011;**2242**(1):9-18. DOI: 10.3141/2242-02

[65] Braithwaite J et al. Health system frameworks and performance indicators in eight countries: A comparative international analysis. SAGE Open Medicine. 2017;**5**:2050312116686516. DOI: 10.1177/2050312116686516

[66] Fekri O, Macarayan ER, Klazinga N. Health System Performance Assessment in the WHO European Region: Which Domains and Indicators have been Used by Member States for its Measurement? Copenhagen: WHO Regional Office for Europe; 2018. [En ligne]. Disponible sur: http://www.ncbi.nlm.nih.gov/books/NBK519096/ [Consulté le: septembre 14, 2020]

Section 5

Care Coordination, Integration, and Social Context

Chapter 7

Practical Care Coordination for Primary Care Providers: Bridging the Gap between Clinical Practice and Patient Outcomes

Daryl O. Traylor, Eboni E. Anderson, Meghan Etsey, Bethany Fenton, Nayla Cheema, Darcy McCampbell, Devki Patel and Brianna Clark

Abstract

Coordinating care effectively lies at the heart of improving patient outcomes, streamlining workflows, and containing costs in primary care. In this setting, primary care providers function as the central communication hub, guiding patients through various services while addressing both clinical needs and the social factors that influence health. In this review, we outline the key pillars of care coordination, patient-focused practices, cross-disciplinary teamwork, and efficient management of health information, and describe practical tactics such as crafting individualized care plans, maximizing electronic health record capabilities, and incorporating telehealth. We also confront systemic hurdles, excessive administrative tasks, disjointed communication channels, and shifting reimbursement schemes, and propose targeted solutions to navigate them. As health systems move toward value-based models, frameworks like patient-centered medical homes and accountable care organizations offer fresh avenues for strengthening coordination. Adopting these innovations enables primary care teams to deliver more cohesive, cost-effective, and patient-driven care.

Keywords: care coordination, primary care provider, interdisciplinary collaboration, health information management, value-based care

1. Introduction

In an era marked by rapidly evolving healthcare landscapes and increasing patient complexity, effective care coordination has emerged as an important cornerstone of quality primary care [1]. This chapter analyzes the core principles that enable primary care clinicians to translate clinical measures into superior patient outcomes. It highlights how a systematic, patient-centered approach, underpinned by robust interdisciplinary collaborations and effective health information management, can transform fragmented care into an integrated, seamless continuum. By examining both the challenges and actionable strategies inherent in care coordination, this chapter highlights the vital role of PCPs as care coordinators and emphasizes the transformative potential of innovations such as electronic health records (EHR), telehealth, and predictive analytics [2]. The chapter challenges PCPs to apply these resources and collaborative models so that every patient receives comprehensive, streamlined, and top-quality care starting with the very first encounter.

1.1 Definition and significance of care coordination

In the primary care setting, care coordination is a means of methodically organizing each aspect of a patient's treatment and keeping all members of the patient care team fully informed [3, 4]. Care coordination principles work to ensure that patient priorities and preferences are identified in advance and promptly relayed to the appropriate team members. This process involves identifying each patient's needs and preferences in advance and making sure they are communicated to the right team members precisely when needed [1].

Effective care coordination is essential in modern healthcare, particularly in primary care settings where providers serve as the initial and central touchpoint for patients. In the absence of coordinated care, patients can end up with disjointed services, avoidable hospital admissions, and repeated testing, all of which drives up costs, reduces trust in their providers, and undermines positive health outcomes [2]. Research has shown that when care coordination is well-organized, it can lower hospital readmissions, enhance chronic disease management, and boost overall patient satisfaction [5–7].

1.2 How primary care providers facilitate care coordination

Primary care providers act as the linchpin of care coordination, serving as the main touchpoint for patients as they navigate the complexities of the healthcare system [8]. Primary care providers are responsible for integrating care across multiple specialists, ensuring that treatment plans are effectively communicated, and advocating for their patients' healthcare needs [1].

In their role as care coordinators, PCPs engage in several key activities [1]:

- Developing and maintaining comprehensive care plans tailored to each patient's medical and social needs.
- Facilitating communication among healthcare providers, including specialists, pharmacists, and mental health professionals.
- Utilizing EHR to track patient progress, laboratory results, and medication adherence.
- Providing patient education and self-management support to promote adherence to prescribed treatments.
- Collaborating with social workers, health navigators, and community health organizations to address social determinants of health that impact patient well-being.

By actively participating in care coordination, PCPs help reduce care fragmentation and ensure a seamless transition between different levels of care [9, 10].

1.3 Care coordination's impact

A robust body of evidence shows that well-coordinated care yields multiple benefits, superior clinical metrics, greater patient satisfaction, and significant reductions in overall costs [2]. Coordinated care reduces the likelihood of medical mistakes, lessens hospital admissions, and improves long-term control of chronic illnesses such as diabetes, high blood pressure, and cardiac disease [5].

Several key benefits of care coordination include [11, 12]:

- *Reduced hospital readmissions*: By ensuring timely follow-up appointments, medication reconciliation, and patient education, care coordination minimizes preventable hospital readmissions.

- *Improved chronic disease management*: Coordinated care facilitates proactive disease monitoring and intervention, leading to better control of chronic conditions and reduced complications.

- *Enhanced patient engagement*: A supportive, well-coordinated care environment fosters stronger adherence to prescribed therapies and motivates patients to engage actively in decisions about their health.

- *Decreased healthcare costs*: By preventing unnecessary emergency room visits, redundant testing, and avoidable hospitalizations, care coordination leads to significant cost savings for healthcare systems and patients alike.

In summary, care coordination is a critical component of primary care practice, bridging the gap between clinical interventions and optimal patient outcomes. By prioritizing collaboration, communication, and patient-centered approaches, PCPs can establish comprehensive, efficient, and high-quality care.

2. Methods

2.1 Research question

This review addresses the following question:

In adult primary care settings, which care coordination strategies—encompassing patient-centered frameworks, interdisciplinary collaboration, health information technologies, and telehealth—are associated with improved patient outcomes?

To structure this inquiry, we adopted a PICO framework:

- *Population (P)*: Adults (≥18 years) receiving care in primary care or family practice settings.

- *Intervention (I)*: Any formal care coordination strategy or model (e.g., patient-centered medical home, interdisciplinary case management, EHR-enabled coordination, telehealth-based follow-up).

- *Comparison (C)*: Usual care or alternative coordination approaches.

- *Outcomes (O)*: Patient-level outcomes (e.g., hospital readmissions, disease control metrics, patient satisfaction, healthcare utilization, cost measures).

2.2 Search strategy

A comprehensive search was conducted in PubMed/MEDLINE, Embase, CINAHL and the Cochrane Library from database inception through May 2025. We supplemented electronic searches by hand-checking reference lists of key articles.

2.2.1 MeSH terms and Boolean operators

The PubMed strategy combined MeSH headings with title/abstract keywords using Boolean logic:

(“Care Coordination”[MeSH Terms]
OR “Patient Care Team”[MeSH Terms]
OR “Case Management”[MeSH Terms]
OR “Patient Navigation”[MeSH Terms])
OR
(“care coordination”[Title/Abstract]
OR “case management”[Title/Abstract]
OR “care management”[Title/Abstract]
OR “patient navigation”[Title/Abstract])
AND
(“Primary Health Care”[Mesh]
OR “Family Practice”[Mesh]
OR “General Practice”[Mesh])
OR
(“primary care”[Title/Abstract]
OR “family medicine”[Title/Abstract]
OR “general practice”[Title/Abstract])
AND
(“Treatment Outcome”[MeSH Terms]
OR “Patient Outcome Assessment”[MeSH Terms]
OR “Hospitalization”[MeSH Terms]
OR “Readmission”[MeSH Terms])
OR
(outcome*[Title/Abstract]
OR readmission*[Title/Abstract]
OR hospitalization*[Title/Abstract]
OR satisfaction[Title/Abstract])
AND
(“Electronic Health Records”[MeSH Terms]
OR “Telemedicine”[MeSH Terms]
OR “Information Systems”[MeSH Terms])
OR
(“EHR”[Title/Abstract]
OR “telehealth”[Title/Abstract]
OR “telemedicine”[Title/Abstract]
OR “health information technolog*”[Title/Abstract])

Search syntax was adapted for each database’s subject headings and field tags.

2.3 Eligibility criteria

Inclusion criteria

1. *Population*: Adults (≥18 years) receiving care in outpatient primary care, family practice, or community health settings.

2. *Intervention*: Any formal or informal care coordination strategy or model (e.g., PCMH, ACO partnerships, interdisciplinary case management, EHR-enabled workflows, telehealth follow-up, patient/navigator–led programs).

3. *Outcomes*: Reports that present quantitative or qualitative data on patient-level outcomes (e.g., hospital readmissions, chronic disease control measures, patient satisfaction, healthcare utilization, cost or efficiency metrics).

Source types:

1. *Peer-reviewed literature*: RCTs, controlled before-after studies, cohort studies, cross-sectional analyses, qualitative inquiries, systematic reviews/meta-analyses, clinical practice guidelines.

2. *Gray literature*: Government and health-system reports, organizational white papers, policy briefs, implementation toolkits, dissertations, full-text conference proceedings.

3. *Language and date*: English-language works published or released between January 2000 and May 2025.

Exclusion criteria

1. Studies conducted exclusively in inpatient, emergency, or specialty settings without a clear primary care component.

2. Pediatric-only populations (<18 years).

3. Sources lacking full-text access (e.g., abstracts without accompanying reports).

4. Publications that did not explicitly evaluate a care coordination strategy or that failed to report patient-level outcomes.

Two reviewers first examined titles and abstracts, and any study deemed potentially relevant was then assessed in full. If the reviewers disagreed at any point, they either resolved the discrepancy through consensus or brought in a third reviewer to decide. From each included study, we recorded details such as the study type, setting, intervention characteristics, outcome measures, and main results to inform a narrative synthesis across the key domains of care coordination.

3. Results

3.1 Study selection

A total of 214 unique records were identified through database searches (PubMed/MEDLINE, Embase, CINAHL, Cochrane Library) and hand-searching of reference lists. After title/abstract screening and full-text review against pre-specified eligibility criteria, 52 sources were retained for synthesis and are listed in the References.

3.2 Characteristics of included sources

- *Study designs*: 15 randomized controlled trials; 10 systematic reviews/meta-analyses; 8 qualitative inquiries; 7 mixed-methods studies; 12 policy reports or gray-literature frameworks.
- *Geographic settings*: Predominantly U.S. (n = 38), with contributions from Canada (n = 5), Europe (n = 6), and low- to middle-income contexts (n = 3).
- *Interventions examined*: Care-coordination models (CCM, PCMH, ACO partnerships), interdisciplinary case-management teams, EHR-enabled workflows, telehealth follow-up, and patient navigation programs.
- *Publication time frame*: 2002–2024, with a notable increase in digital-health and telehealth studies after 2015.

3.3 Synthesis of key findings

1. Patient-centered frameworks
   - Models such as the Chronic Care Model [1] and patient-centered medical homes consistently demonstrated reductions in hospital readmissions [5] and improved chronic-disease metrics [3].
2. Interdisciplinary collaboration
   - Team-based approaches, involving physicians, nurses, pharmacists, social workers, and navigators, were associated with higher patient satisfaction scores and enhanced engagement in self-management [8, 13].
3. Health information management
   - EHR-Enabled Coordination reduced duplicative testing and improved medication reconciliation [14, 15]. Predictive analytics embedded within EHRs facilitated early identification of high-risk patients [16].
   - Telehealth and Remote Monitoring increased access for rural and underserved populations, with virtual follow-up linked to lower readmission rates and timely detection of clinical deteriorations [17, 18].
4. Care transitions
   - Structured discharge protocols and transitional-care interventions (e.g., Coleman's Care Transitions Intervention) significantly reduced 30-day readmissions and improved continuity between hospital and primary care.
5. Gaps and underexplored areas
   - Heterogeneity in outcome measures: Lack of standardized metrics hampers cross-study comparisons.

DOI: http://dx.doi.org/10.5772/intechopen.1011662

- Equity and social determinants: Few studies systematically examine how coordination strategies address housing, food insecurity, or cultural competence.
- Long-term cost-effectiveness: Evidence on sustained financial impact remains limited beyond 12-month follow-up.
- Rural and resource-constrained settings: Underrepresentation in the literature, despite unique coordination challenges.

4. Core principles of effective care coordination

At its core, effective care coordination is built on a philosophy that places patients at the center of every decision, ensuring that care is as unique and dynamic as the individuals it serves [8]. Rather than imposing inflexible rules, the aim is to cultivate a clinical setting in which patients are genuinely listened to, respected, and meaningfully participatory in shaping their own care. It invites a dialog that bridges clinical expertise with personal experience, allowing for decisions that respect the diverse cultural, social, and economic backgrounds of patients [13].

In parallel, a seamless healthcare experience is realized through the collective efforts of a dedicated team of professionals. When the unique expertise of physicians, nurses, social workers, pharmacists, and care navigators is harnessed collectively, care coordination becomes a joint obligation, one that dissolves professional silos to provide seamless, comprehensive support [13]. Together, these collaborative efforts foster an environment of clear communication and mutual accountability, ensuring that each patient receives care that is effective, compassionate, and personalized.

This section explains these fundamental principles, illustrating how an organic blend of patient-centered care and interdisciplinary collaboration can transform fragmented healthcare into a unified, responsive, and deeply human system.

4.1 Patient-centered approach: Care coordination frameworks

A patient-centered approach is the foundation of effective care coordination, affirming that healthcare services align with individual patient needs, preferences, and values [8]. This model emphasizes active patient involvement in healthcare decisions, fostering trust and engagement between patients and providers. When candid dialog and joint decision-making take center stage, patient-focused care cultivates greater satisfaction, more consistent adherence to prescribed therapies, and measurably improved health outcomes [2]. Moreover, it facilitates collaboration among multidisciplinary teams, enabling more holistic, personalized care that is tailored to each individual's unique medical and social context [13]. Rooted in these guiding tenets, modern care-coordination models now function as indispensable mechanisms for aligning and synchronizing services along the entire continuum of care. They are particularly vital for patients facing chronic or multifaceted conditions, ensuring that health systems operate not only with efficiency but with an authentic responsiveness to each individual's lived experience.

A care coordination framework is a structured, strategic approach designed to streamline and integrate patient care activities across various healthcare providers, disciplines, and settings [19, 20]. Its central aim is to ensure that patients, particularly those with complex, chronic, or high-risk health conditions, receive comprehensive, person-centered, and efficient care throughout the continuum of services [21]. As the healthcare landscape increasingly emphasizes value-based care, such frameworks have become essential tools in promoting continuity, safety, and effectiveness in service delivery.

At the heart of any care coordination framework lies the principle of patient-centered care. This element places the individual's preferences, values, needs, and life goals at the core of decision-making processes [2, 8]. Patients, and when appropriate, their relatives, should be recognized as collaborative architects and co-executors of the care strategy. A truly effective framework recognizes that clinical interventions are most successful when aligned with the patient's lived experiences and social realities.

Another foundational component is the interdisciplinary team-based approach, which fosters collaboration among physicians, nurses, case managers, pharmacists, social workers, and other health professionals [13]. This collaborative team design encourages transparent communication, clearly defined responsibilities, and collective accountability, guaranteeing that each dimension of a patient's wellbeing, clinical, psychosocial, behavioral, and environmental, is managed in a unified, coordinated fashion. Care planning serves as the operational backbone of coordinated care. Individualized care plans, grounded in evidence-based practices, are developed with measurable goals and routinely updated to reflect changes in the patient's condition or social context [19]. These plans become living documents that guide the patient journey across multiple encounters and care settings.

Equally critical is information sharing and communication, which enables timely, accurate, and bidirectional exchange of patient information. The deliberate integration of health IT, encompassing electronic health records, clinical decision-support tools, and encrypted messaging, keeps the entire care team thoroughly informed and aligned in its clinical choices [4].

Transition management addresses the vulnerabilities that arise during shifts between care settings, such as hospital discharge or specialist referral [22]. This component emphasizes continuity and safety, aiming to reduce duplication of services, medication discrepancies, and unnecessary readmissions. Linked to this is monitoring and follow-up, which entails the regular assessment of a patient's progress, adherence to treatment, and evolving needs [23]. Through proactive outreach and surveillance, the care team can intervene early and adjust care plans as needed.

Finally, measurement and accountability ensure that care coordination efforts are producing meaningful results. Most frameworks monitor a core set of performance metrics: patient satisfaction ratings, outcome measures, rehospitalization frequencies, and cost benchmarks [23]. Insights from these data fuel continuous quality improvement and uphold organizational transparency and accountability.

Several well-established models illustrate the principles and application of care coordination frameworks [24, 25]. The Agency for Healthcare Research and Quality (AHRQ) framework, for instance, categorizes core coordination activities, such as communication and medication management, around patient needs and system-level enablers. The Chronic Care Model (CCM) advocates for empowered patients and proactive clinical teams, focusing on redesigning care processes to support long-term disease management. The Patient-Centered Medical Home (PCMH) operates as a primary-care-anchored model that weaves behavioral health, social support, and specialty services into one coherent, continuous system of care.

The adoption of care coordination frameworks has demonstrated considerable value in health care [21]. When implemented effectively, they reduce preventable medical errors and adverse events, improve clinical outcomes for patients with multiple chronic conditions, and foster higher levels of patient engagement and satisfaction. Additionally, these frameworks can contribute to cost containment by minimizing redundant services and improving resource allocation. In an era of increasing complexity and constrained resources, care coordination frameworks represent both a moral imperative and a strategic necessity for modern health systems.

4.1.1 Patient: Family co-decision-making

When patients and their families actively participate in choosing care options, adherence to prescribed therapies increases and health results are more favorable [13]. Providers must foster open communication, encourage patient participation, and consider cultural, social, and economic factors that influence healthcare choices. Strategies include motivational interviewing, goal-setting, and active listening to enhance patient engagement [20].

4.1.2 Shared decision-making and health literacy

Shared decision-making (SDM) blends clinician expertise with each patient's expressed priorities, empowering individuals to select their course of care based on well-informed judgment [21]. Health literacy plays a critical role in this process, as patients must understand medical information to make sound decisions [21]. Clinicians can heighten patient comprehension and agency by adopting clear, jargon-free language, supplementing explanations with visual tools, and confirming understanding via teach-back techniques.

4.2 Interdisciplinary collaboration

Care coordination is most effective when healthcare professionals work collaboratively within an interdisciplinary team [13]. Each team member brings unique expertise, contributing to holistic and comprehensive patient care. Effective interdisciplinary collaboration enhances communication, reduces care fragmentation, and ultimately improves patient outcomes and satisfaction [13]. By leveraging diverse perspectives, healthcare teams can proactively address patient needs and reduce the likelihood of medical errors.

4.2.1 Roles and responsibilities of different healthcare professionals

Interdisciplinary healthcare teams are composed of professionals from diverse clinical and non-clinical backgrounds, each contributing specialized expertise to support holistic, patient-centered care. By clearly defining roles and fostering collaborative engagement, such teams can address complex patient needs more comprehensively, reduce redundancies, and enhance health outcomes [23]. The effectiveness of an interdisciplinary approach hinges on mutual respect, coordinated efforts, and a shared commitment to optimizing patient well-being.

Key roles within the team include:

- *Physicians* serve as primary diagnosticians and clinical decision-makers. They assess symptoms, order and interpret diagnostic tests, formulate medical diagnoses, and establish evidence-based treatment plans. Physicians also collaborate with other providers to adapt care based on clinical progress and evolving patient needs.

- *Nurses* are essential in translating medical plans into practice. Their responsibilities include administering medications and treatments, monitoring vital signs and patient responses, providing education on disease management and health promotion, and serving as patient advocates. Nurses often act as the first point of contact, making them integral to continuity of care and early identification of complications.

- *Social workers* address the psychosocial, emotional, and environmental factors affecting patient health. They conduct psychosocial assessments, provide counseling, assist in advance care planning, and connect patients with essential social services, such as housing, transportation, or financial assistance. Social workers are particularly critical in managing social determinants of health and ensuring equitable care.

- *Pharmacists* bring specialized knowledge in pharmacotherapy. Key duties include systematically scrutinizing medication regimens to verify safety, therapeutic efficacy, and potential interactions; educating patients on correct drug use; and collaborating with prescribers to maximize treatment success. Pharmacists also play a vital role in promoting adherence and reducing medication-related error.

- *Health navigators and community health workers* (also known as patient navigators or care coordinators) assist patients in understanding and accessing the healthcare system. They guide patients through complex processes such as referrals, insurance coverage, and appointment scheduling, while addressing logistical and cultural barriers to care. Navigators enhance patient engagement and help reduce delays in treatment.

Together, these professionals form an integrated network wherein each role complements the others, enabling a seamless continuum of care. Clearly delineated responsibilities, open communication, and coordinated workflows ensure that care is both efficient and responsive to the multidimensional needs of patients.

4.2.2 Building an effective care team

Establishing a well-functioning care team requires clear communication, defined roles, and shared accountability [23, 24]. Regular interdisciplinary meetings, case conferences, and collaborative care models improve coordination and patient outcomes [24]. Utilizing standardized protocols and leveraging team-based care principles enhances efficiency and effectiveness.

4.3 Health information management

In today's interconnected healthcare landscape, health information management (HIM) is a vital thread that weaves together every facet of patient care. The seamless integration of digital tools has transformed the way healthcare providers access and share critical patient information and has ensured that clinical decision-making is informed by real-time data [25, 26]. By leveraging technologies such as EHR and telehealth solutions, care teams can streamline transitions, monitor progress, and manage chronic conditions more effectively [25]. This HIM not only minimizes redundant efforts and enhances decision-making but also extends quality care to underserved communities, breaking down traditional barriers to access. Ultimately, robust HIM empowers providers to deliver care that is both timely and tailored to the individual needs of each patient, fostering a more efficient and responsive healthcare system [25, 26].

4.3.1 Utilizing electronic health records (EHRs) for coordinated care

Electronic health records give clinicians instantaneous visibility into a patient's past medical narrative, current laboratory findings, and active care plans, curtailing redundant work and sharpening clinical decisions [27]. Effective use of EHR supports better care transitions, medication reconciliation, and chronic disease management. Additionally, EHR can facilitate improved communication among interdisciplinary care teams, promoting coordinated care and patient safety [28]. Moreover, EHR enhances clinical efficiency by integrating clinical decision support tools, automating routine administrative tasks, and enabling data analytics for population health management [28, 29]. By leveraging predictive analytics and artificial intelligence (AI), EHR can help identify at-risk patients, optimize treatment plans, and support evidence-based practice, ultimately improving health outcomes and reducing healthcare costs.

4.3.2 Virtual care and remote monitoring

Virtual consultation platforms and remote monitoring technologies have fundamentally reshaped care coordination, granting clinicians immediate reach and support for individuals—most notably those in rural or otherwise resource-limited communities [30]. These technologies allow providers to monitor patient progress, conduct virtual consultations, and enhance patient engagement, while reducing the burden on in-person healthcare facilities [30, 31]. Furthermore, telehealth solutions support timely interventions and improve clinical outcomes by enabling earlier detection of potential health issues [31]. By integrating telehealth into routine care delivery, healthcare systems can reduce disparities and promote equitable access to essential health services.

5. Strategies for enhancing care coordination

Effective care coordination thrives on the creation and continual refinement of personalized care plans that serve as both a roadmap and a living document for patient care [14, 17]. At the heart of these strategies is the commitment to develop plans that integrate detailed patient histories, clearly defined treatment goals, and thoughtfully tailored interventions, ensuring that every step of care is purposeful and aligned with the patient's unique circumstances [2]. Such plans are not static; they evolve through ongoing monitoring and adjustments based on real-world outcomes and feedback. This dynamic process not only helps with transitions across different care settings but also addresses the broader spectrum of medical and social determinants, ultimately enhancing patient engagement, adherence, and overall health outcomes.

5.1 Designing and executing care strategies

Developing and implementing care plans is a cornerstone of effective care coordination, a dynamic process that transforms clinical data and patient narratives into actionable, personalized roadmaps for health [2]. The process begins by building a holistic profile that includes the patient's medical background, therapeutic objectives, and current challenges, guaranteeing that all elements of care, from clinical interventions to relevant social determinants, are fully integrated [15]. These care plans are then meticulously tailored to resonate with individual patient preferences, cultural contexts, and unique life circumstances, fostering a sense of ownership and engagement in the care journey.

Beyond their initial creation, care plans are living documents that evolve in response to ongoing assessments and patient progress [16]. Regular reviews and adjustments, driven by feedback from both the patient and the interdisciplinary care team, ensure that the care plan remains relevant and effective over time. This continuous refinement can bridge the gaps in care and propel the overall system toward a more responsive, integrated, and patient-centered model of healthcare delivery.

5.1.1 Key components of a comprehensive care plan

A well-structured care plan includes patient history, treatment goals, prescribed interventions, and monitoring strategies. It safeguards continuity of care and addresses both medical and social determinants of health [15, 16]. Incorporating patient preferences and active participation in care planning further enhances adherence and promotes personalized care delivery. Additionally, regularly updating and clearly communicating care plans among interdisciplinary team members strengthens collaboration and provides alignment with evolving patient needs.

Specifically, a comprehensive care plan should include the following components [18, 32, 33]:

- *Patient demographics and history*: Includes age, gender, cultural background, medical history, previous diagnoses, allergies, medications, and relevant family history.

- *Assessment and diagnostic information*: Results of recent physical examinations, diagnostic tests, imaging, and laboratory findings.

- *Individualized treatment goals*: Clearly defined, measurable, achievable goals that reflect patient preferences, clinical needs, and desired health outcomes.

- *Prescribed interventions*: Detailed descriptions of recommended treatments, therapies, medications, and lifestyle modifications tailored to patient-specific conditions.

- *Monitoring and evaluation strategies*: Methods and timelines for assessing patient progress, treatment efficacy, medication adherence, and early detection of complications.

- *Patient education and self-care management*: Information and resources are provided to patients to support understanding of their condition, adherence to the care plan, and proactive health management.

- *Social determinants of health*: Identification and strategies to address social factors such as housing, nutrition, transportation, employment status, and community support systems.

- *Care coordination and communication plan*: Clearly outlined team duties, robust communication channels, and methods for smooth handoffs across care settings.

Ultimately, the comprehensive care plan functions not merely as a document, but as a dynamic framework that drives collaborative, patient-centered practice. Regular updates and clear dissemination across the care team are essential to maintaining alignment with the patient's evolving needs and to ensuring seamless, integrated care delivery.

5.1.2 Customizing care plans to meet individual patient needs

Personalized care plans thoughtfully integrate patient preferences, cultural backgrounds, values, and social circumstances, establishing trust and enhancing patient-provider relationships. This tailored approach promotes greater patient engagement, improves adherence to recommended interventions, and, in time, contributes to superior clinical outcomes. Furthermore, by addressing individual barriers and leveraging unique patient strengths, personalized care plans support health equity and empower patients in their own health management [16]. In doing so, personalized care plans elevate the quality of care and transform the healthcare experience into one that is truly collaborative, responsive, and patient-centered.

5.1.3 Monitoring and adjusting care plans over time

Care plans should be dynamic, incorporating regular assessments and timely modifications guided by patient progress, evolving clinical conditions, and collaborative feedback from interdisciplinary care teams [15, 16, 18, 32, 33]. Consistent monitoring enables the early identification of treatment inefficiencies or emerging health issues, facilitating proactive adjustments to interventions. Continuous communication among healthcare providers, patients, and caregivers further guarantees that care plans remain responsive, patient-centered, and aligned with current clinical evidence and patient preferences.

6. Challenges in care coordination and practical solutions

Care coordination stands at the heart of high-performing healthcare systems, yet its successful implementation remains elusive in many clinical settings. Although coordinated care is vital for elevating patient outcomes and optimizing service delivery, initiatives to establish it routinely face considerable barriers. Providers must navigate a complex system of policies, administrative burdens, and systemic inefficiencies that create substantial barriers to effective collaboration and patient-centered care. From regulatory constraints to evolving reimbursement models, these challenges require innovative, strategic solutions that balance compliance with the need for efficiency and accessibility.

Addressing these hurdles is not just about overcoming obstacles; it is about reimagining workflows, enhancing communication, and leveraging policy changes to create a healthcare system that is structured and adaptable. Achieving this vision demands a unified commitment across all levels of healthcare, from frontline clinicians to policymakers, to invest in integrated infrastructure, champion cross-sector collaboration, and embed flexibility into system design. By identifying and tackling these challenges head-on, PCPs can drive meaningful improvements in coordination, ascertaining that patient care remains seamless, equitable, and sustainable.

6.1 Regulatory and policy challenges

The intersection of healthcare policy and care coordination is both intricate and influential, shaping how providers communicate, share data, and manage care transitions. Regulatory frameworks, while essential for maintaining patient privacy and standardizing care delivery, can also introduce complexities that hinder seamless coordination [34]. Understanding and complying with these policies is essential to ensuring that care remains both legally sound and patient centered.

Additionally, the healthcare reimbursement landscape is shifting from traditional fee-for-service models to value-based care initiatives that incentivize quality over quantity [35, 36]. While these models encourage more integrated, outcome-driven care, they also require significant investment in data management, workflow optimization, and technological infrastructure [25, 37]. Providers must adapt to these evolving financial structures, while maintaining a focus on patient needs to ensure that the push for cost efficiency does not compromise care quality. Successfully navigating these regulatory and reimbursement challenges is vitally important for creating a coordinated care system that is financially viable and clinically effective.

6.1.1 Navigating healthcare policies affecting care coordination

Healthcare policies exert a profound influence on the design and execution of care coordination strategies. Regulatory frameworks governing patient privacy, data interoperability, and reimbursement structures directly shape the ways in which healthcare providers exchange information, engage in interdisciplinary collaboration, and deliver integrated services [38, 39]. Successfully navigating today's intricate policy environment demands a thorough command of both federal and state requirements, chief among them the Affordable Care Act, HIPAA provisions, and Centers for Medicare and Medicaid Services (CMS) directives [40, 41]. To optimize patient outcomes, healthcare professionals must adeptly balance regulatory compliance with the implementation of streamlined, patient-centered coordination practices that promote continuity of care, reduce redundancies, and enhance the overall quality and efficiency of service delivery [41].

6.1.2 Aligning with value-based payment models

The transition from fee-for-service reimbursement to value-based payment models creates fresh possibilities for stronger care coordination while also introducing new complexities. Payment models, including the Merit-Based Incentive Payment System (MIPS) and accountable care organizations (ACOs), reward providers for delivering well-coordinated, high-quality care [42]. However, adapting to these models requires investment in health information technology, data analytics, and workflow redesign to meet performance metrics and safeguard financial sustainability [43]. Moreover, successful integration demands strong leadership, interprofessional collaboration, and continuous quality improvement processes to align clinical practice with evolving reimbursement structures. Without these foundational supports, organizations risk misalignment between care coordination goals and financial incentives, potentially undermining both patient outcomes and organizational viability.

6.2 Systemic barriers to effective coordination

Systemic barriers can undermine even the most well-intentioned efforts to coordinate care, creating obstacles that impede the smooth flow of information and services [25]. In many healthcare settings, inefficient workflows and overwhelming administrative tasks not only slow down processes but also divert valuable time and energy away from patient-centered care. Similarly, communication gaps often rooted in fragmented systems and isolated data silos, can lead to critical information being overlooked, compromising the continuity and quality of care [25]. By recognizing and addressing these challenges, healthcare organizations can streamline operations and foster an environment where clear, consistent communication supports every step of the patient journey.

6.2.1 Workflow inefficiencies and administrative burdens

Many healthcare organizations struggle with inefficient workflows that hinder effective care coordination. Excessive documentation requirements, redundant administrative tasks, and lack of standardized processes create barriers to seamless communication and care transitions [44]. Streamlining workflows through automation, reducing unnecessary paperwork, and integrating clinical decision support tools can improve efficiency and allow providers to focus more on patient-centered care. By doing so, healthcare teams are better positioned to prioritize clinical judgment, improve interdisciplinary collaboration, and devote more time to delivering personalized, patient-centered care that improves outcomes and satisfaction.

6.2.2 Communication gaps among healthcare providers

Effective communication is a cornerstone of successful care coordination, serving as the foundation for timely, safe, and patient-centered care. However, many healthcare systems continue to experience substantial breakdowns in provider-to-provider communication. Inconsistencies in clinical documentation, reliance on siloed EHR systems, and limited interoperability between disparate health information systems significantly compromise the continuity and quality of care [45]. These communication failures can lead to redundant testing, medication errors, delayed interventions, and poor patient outcomes, particularly during transitions of care [46]. To mitigate these risks, healthcare organizations must prioritize the adoption of standardized handoff protocols, implement interoperable EHR systems that support real-time data exchange, and foster a culture of collaborative communication across multidisciplinary teams. Strengthening these communication pathways can enhance care coordination and improve clinical efficiency, patient satisfaction, and health systems performance.

6.3 Overcoming common obstacles

Overcoming obstacles in care coordination demands a multifaceted approach that combines enhanced communication with the smart use of technology. By fostering interprofessional dialog through structured tools, regular team meetings, and dedicated training programs, healthcare teams can break down silos and provide vital patient information that is consistently shared [13, 26]. At the same time, leveraging advancements in digital health, such as interoperable EHR systems, telehealth platforms, and AI-powered decision support tools, paves the way for a more integrated and efficient care delivery system [47]. Together, these strategies can address common challenges and empower providers to deliver care that is collaborative and patient-focused, eventually leading to improved outcomes and a more resilient healthcare system.

6.3.1 Solutions for improving interprofessional communication

Interprofessional collaboration is essential for effective care coordination. Strategies for improving communication among healthcare professionals include [48, 49]:

- Adopting formalized communication frameworks, exemplified by the SBAR (Situation–Background–Assessment–Recommendation) method, and deploying standardized clinical pathways.

- Conducting routine multidisciplinary meetings to review patient cases and align care strategies.

- Utilizing secure and encrypted messaging platforms that facilitate real-time communication between care team members.

- Providing interprofessional training programs to enhance team-based problem-solving and collaboration skills.

By integrating these strategies into routine practice, healthcare organizations can move toward a model of coordinated, high-quality care where communication is intentional, inclusive, and centered on optimizing patient outcomes.

6.3.2 Implementing technology-driven coordination tools

Advancements in health technology have revolutionized care coordination. Key technology-driven solutions include [50, 51]:

- Enhanced EHR interoperability allows seamless information exchange across healthcare settings.

- Telehealth platforms provide remote consultations and real-time patient monitoring to improve access to care.

- Via patient portals, people can book appointments, review their laboratory results, and correspond directly with their clinicians.

- AI-powered decision support tools assist clinicians in making data-driven treatment decisions.

By surmounting regulatory hurdles, streamlining operational processes, fostering clear communication, and harnessing modern technology, healthcare systems can refine care coordination and, ultimately, achieve superior patient outcomes.

7. Conclusion

In wrapping up the exploration of care coordination, this chapter focuses on its vital role in delivering seamless, integrated care across all healthcare settings. The concluding section summarizes the core insights and takeaways for PCPs. Additionally, this section charts a clear path forward, emphasizing actionable strategies and visionary perspectives for the future of primary care coordination.

7.1 Summary of key takeaways for primary care providers

Effective care coordination is a cornerstone of high-quality primary care, which asserts that patients receive seamless, integrated services across healthcare settings. Primary care providers play a pivotal role in orchestrating communication, managing interdisciplinary collaboration, and leveraging technology to improve care transitions [1, 8]. While systemic challenges such as administrative burdens, fragmented communication, and shifting reimbursement models persist, targeted strategies can mitigate these obstacles [52]. By implementing structured communication tools, enhancing interprofessional teamwork, and optimizing health information technology, PCPs can significantly enhance patient engagement, reduce hospitalizations, and improve chronic disease management.

7.2 Daily care coordination: Action steps

To enhance care coordination in everyday clinical practice, PCPs must adopt a multifaceted, evidence-based approach that integrates communication, technology, personalized care, interdisciplinary collaboration, and advocacy. One critical component is improving interprofessional communication using standardized handoff frameworks, such as SBAR, along with holding regular interdisciplinary meetings to ensure all care team members are aligned on treatment goals. Technological solutions should also be leveraged; optimizing EHR interoperability, integrating telehealth services, and utilizing secure messaging platforms can facilitate timely and accurate information sharing among providers.

Equally important is the development of individualized, patient-centered care plans that consider not only clinical conditions but also the social determinants of health, cultural values, and the availability of support systems. This level of personalization can increase patient engagement and adherence, while improving care outcomes. Furthermore, strengthening collaboration across disciplines by actively involving specialists, pharmacists, social workers, and community health worker/health navigators can assure that care is comprehensive and coordinated across all points of service.

Lastly, PCPs should engage in efforts to influence systemic and policy-level changes. This includes advocating for reforms that reduce administrative burden, support adequate reimbursement for care coordination activities, and promote sustainable models of integrated care. By embedding these strategies into routine practice, PCPs are positioned to significantly improve the quality, efficiency, and equity of healthcare delivery.

7.3 Primary care coordination: Emerging models and opportunities

The future of care coordination in primary care will be shaped by technological advancements, evolving healthcare delivery models, and policy-driven reimbursement reforms. Integrating AI-powered decision aids, prognostic data analytics, and continuous remote monitoring is poised to strengthen anticipatory, patient-tailored care models. As payment structures transition to value-driven models, exemplified by patient-centered medical homes (PCMH) and ACOs, they increasingly amplify incentives for integrated, well-coordinated, and holistic patient management.

As these models evolve, PCPs must remain adaptable, embracing innovative tools and interdisciplinary collaboration to optimize patient-centered care. The time to act is now: PCPs must position themselves as leaders in driving systemic change by championing innovation, influencing policy reform, and prioritizing equity in care delivery. By leveraging emerging opportunities and advocating for systemic improvements, PCPs can lead the way in shaping a more efficient, equitable, and sustainable healthcare system.

Conflict of interest

The authors declare no conflict of interest.

Author details

Daryl O. Traylor[1*], Eboni E. Anderson[2], Meghan Etsey[3], Bethany Fenton[3], Nayla Cheema[2], Darcy McCampbell[4], Devki Patel[5] and Brianna Clark[6]

1 Oceania University of Medicine, Apia, Samoa

2 A.T. Still University School of Osteopathic Medicine in Arizona, Mesa, AZ, United States

3 St. George's University School of Medicine, St. George's, Grenada

4 Eastern Washington University, Cheney, WA, United States

5 Texas Tech University Health Sciences Center School of Medicine, Lubbock, TX, United States

6 Sunflower Lactation and Health Education LLC, Joplin, MO, United States

*Address all correspondence to: daryl.traylor@oum.edu.ws

References

[1] Bodenheimer T, Wagner EH, Grumbach K. Improving primary care for patients with chronic illness: The chronic care model, part 2. Journal of the American Medical Association. 2002;**288**(14):1775-1779. DOI: 10.1001/jama.288.15.1909

[2] Coleman EA, Parry C, Chalmers S, Min SJ. The care transitions intervention: Results of a randomized controlled trial. Archives of Internal Medicine. 2006;**166**(17):1822-1828. DOI: 10.1001/archinte.166.17.1822

[3] McDonald KM, Sundaram V, Bravata DM, et al. Closing the Quality Gap: A Critical Analysis of Quality Improvement Strategies (Vol. 7: Care Coordination). Rockville (MD): Agency for Healthcare Research and Quality (US); 2007 (Technical Reviews, No. 9.7.). Available from: https://www.ncbi.nlm.nih.gov/books/NBK44015/

[4] Stille CJ, Jerant A, Bell D, Meltzer D, Elmore JG. Coordinating care across diseases, settings, and clinicians: A key role for the generalist in practice. Annals of Internal Medicine. 2005;**142**(8):700-708. DOI: 10.7326/0003-4819-142-8-200504190-00038

[5] Peikes D, Chen A, Schore J, Brown R. Effects of care coordination on hospitalization, quality of care, and health care expenditures among Medicare beneficiaries: 15 randomized trials. Journal of the American Medical Association. 2009;**301**(6):603-618. DOI: 10.1001/jama.2009.126

[6] Wang MC, Mosen D, Shuster E, Bellows J. Association of patient-reported care coordination with patient satisfaction. The Journal of Ambulatory Care Management. 2015;**38**(1):69-76. DOI: 10.1097/JAC.0000000000000021

[7] McCarthy D, Cohen A, Johnson MB. Gaining Ground: Care Management Programs to Reduce Hospital Admissions and Readmissions among Chronically Ill and Vulnerable Patients [Internet]. New York (NY): Commonwealth Fund; 2013. Available from: https://www.commonwealthfund.org/publications/case-study/2013/jan/gaining-ground-care-management-programs-reduce-hospital-admissions [Accessed: March 22, 2025]

[8] Epstein RM, Street RL. The values and value of patient-centered care. Annals of Family Medicine. 2011;**9**(2):100-103. DOI: 10.1370/afm.1239

[9] Lockhart E, Hawker GA, Ivers NM, O'Brien T, Mukerji G, Pariser P, et al. Engaging primary care physicians in care coordination for patients with complex medical conditions. Canadian Family Physician. 2019;**65**(4):e155-e162

[10] Jones CD, Vu MB, O'Donnell CM, Anderson ME, Patel S, Wald HL, et al. A failure to communicate: A qualitative exploration of care coordination between hospitalists and primary care providers around patient hospitalizations. Journal of General Internal Medicine. 2015;**30**(4):417-424. DOI: 10.1007/s11606-014-3056-x

[11] Chang GM, Tung YC. Impact of care coordination on 30-day readmission, mortality, and costs for heart failure. The American Journal of Managed Care. 2024;**30**(4):e116-e123. DOI: 10.37765/ajmc.2024.89533

[12] Chen CC, Cheng SH. Care continuity and care coordination: A preliminary

examination of their effects on hospitalization. Medical Care Research and Review. 2021;**78**(5):475-489. DOI: 10.1177/1077558720903882

[13] Mitchell P, Wynia M, Golden R, McNellis B, Okun S, Webb CE, et al. Core Principles and Values of Effective Team-Based Health Care [Internet]. Washington (DC): Institute of Medicine of the National Academies; 2012. Available from: https://nam.edu/wp-content/uploads/2015/06/VSRT-Team-Based-Care-Principles-Values.pdf [Accessed: March 22, 2025]

[14] Adeniyi AO, Arowoogun JO, Chidi R, Okolo CA, Babawarun O. The impact of electronic health records on patient care and outcomes: A comprehensive review. World Journal of Advanced Research and Reviews. 2024;**21**(2):1446-1455. DOI: 10.30574/wjarr.2024.21.2.0592

[15] Silow-Carroll S, Edwards JN, Rodin D. Using electronic health records to improve quality and efficiency: The experiences of leading hospitals. Issue Brief (Commonwealth Fund). 2012;**17**:1-40. Available from: https://www.commonwealthfund.org/sites/default/files/documents/___media_files_publications_issue_brief_2012_jul_1608_silowcarroll_using_ehrs_improve_quality.pdf

[16] Rao S, Brammer C, McKethan A, Buntin MB. Health information technology: Transforming chronic disease management and care transitions. Primary Care. 2012;**39**(2):327-344. DOI: 10.1016/j.pop.2012.03.006

[17] Kvedar J, Coye MJ, Everett W. Connected health: A review of technologies and strategies to improve patient care with telemedicine and telehealth. Health Affairs. 2014;**33**(2):194-199. DOI: 10.1377/hlthaff.2013.0992

[18] Vudathaneni VKP, Lanke RB, Mudaliyar MC, Movva KV, Kalluri LM, Boyapati R. The impact of telemedicine and remote patient monitoring on healthcare delivery: A comprehensive evaluation. Cureus. 2024;**16**(3):e55534. DOI: 10.7759/cureus.55534

[19] Mosher D. A framework for patient-centred care coordination [article in English, French]. Healthcare Management Forum. 2014;**27**(Suppl. 1):S37-S45. DOI: 10.1016/j.hcmf.2014.01.004

[20] Colombani F, Encrenaz G, Sibé M, Quintard B, Ravaud A, Saillour-Glénisson F, et al. Development of an evidence-based reference framework for care coordination with a focus on the micro level of integrated care: A mixed method design study combining scoping review of reviews and nominal group technique. Health Policy. 2022;**126**(3):245-261. DOI: 10.1016/j.healthpol.2022.01.003

[21] Peterson K, Anderson J, Bourne D, Charns MP, Sheinfeld Gorin S, Hynes DM, et al. Health care coordination theoretical frameworks: A systematic scoping review to increase their understanding and use in practice. Journal of General Internal Medicine. 2019;**34**(Suppl. 1):90-98. DOI: 10.1007/s11606-019-04966-z

[22] Boling PA. Care transitions and home health care. Clinics in Geriatric Medicine. 2009;**25**(1):135-148, viii. DOI: 10.1016/j.cger.2008.11.005

[23] Naylor MD, Shaid EC, Carpenter D, Gass B, Levine C, Li J, et al. Components of comprehensive and effective transitional care. Journal of the American Geriatrics Society. 2017;**65**(6):1119-1125. DOI: 10.1111/jgs.14782

[24] McPheters ML, Kripalani S, Peterson NB, Idowu RT, Jerome RN,

Potter SA, et al. Closing the quality gap: Revisiting the state of the science (vol 3: Quality improvement interventions to address health disparities). Evidence Report/Technology Assessment (Full Rep). 2012 Aug;(208.3):1-475

[25] Van Houdt S, Heyrman J, Vanhaecht K, Sermeus W, De Lepeleire J. An in-depth analysis of theoretical frameworks for the study of care coordination. International Journal of Integrated Care. 2013;**13**:e024. DOI: 10.5334/ijic.1068

[26] Katz DA, Wu C, Jaske E, Stewart GL, Mohr DC. Care practices to promote patient engagement in VA primary care: Factors associated with high performance. Annals of Family Medicine. 2020;**18**(5):397-405. DOI: 10.1370/afm.2569

[27] Liu Y, Wamkpah NS, Ballamudi A, Spataro E, Branham G, Nguyen D, et al. Shared decision-making in patients seeking surgery for facial trauma: The role of decisional conflict and perceived discrimination. Facial Plastic Surgery and Aesthetic Medicine. 2024;**26**(3):333-338. DOI: 10.1089/fpsam.2023.0182

[28] Muscat DM, Shepherd HL, Nutbeam D, Trevena L, McCaffery KJ. Health literacy and shared decision-making: Exploring the relationship to enable meaningful patient engagement in healthcare. Journal of General Internal Medicine. 2021;**36**(2):521-524. DOI: 10.1007/s11606-020-05912-0

[29] Schrager S. Focus on team-based care. WMJ: Official Publication of the State Medical Society of Wisconsin. 2020;**119**(3):149-148. Available from: https://wmjonline.org/wp-content/uploads/2020/119/3/149.pdf

[30] Spitzer EG, Kaitz J, Fix GM, Harvey KLL, Stadnick NA, Sullivan JL, et al. Developing relational coordination: A qualitative study of outpatient mental health teams. Administration and Policy in Mental Health. 2023;**50**(4):591-602. DOI: 10.1007/s10488-023-01261-2

[31] Buntin MB, Burke MF, Hoaglin MC, Blumenthal D. The benefits of health information technology: A review of the recent literature shows predominantly positive results. Health Affairs. 2011;**30**(3):464-471. DOI: 10.1377/hlthaff.2011.0178

[32] Chandrakar M. Revolutionizing rural health care: The power of telehealth and digital health literacy. Current Medical Issues. 2024;**22**(4):255-258. DOI: 10.4103/cmi.cmi_50_24

[33] Edwards ST, Dorr DA, Landon BE. Can personalized care planning improve primary care? Journal of the American Medical Association. 2017;**318**(1):25-26. DOI: 10.1001/jama.2017.6953

[34] Lion KC, Mangione-Smith R, Britto MT. Individualized plans of care to improve outcomes among children and adults with chronic illness: A systematic review. Care Management Journals. 2014;**15**(1):11-25. DOI: 10.1891/1521-0987.15.1.11

[35] Johansson B, Harkey J. Care coordination in long-term home- and community-based care. Home Healthcare Nurse. 2014;**32**(8):470-475. DOI: 10.1097/NHH.0000000000000126

[36] Theodorou ME, Henschen BL, Chapman M. The comprehensive care plan: A patient-centered, multidisciplinary communication tool for frequently hospitalized patients. Joint Commission Journal on Quality and Patient Safety. 2020;**46**(4):217-226. DOI: 10.1016/j.jcjq.2020.01.002

[37] Walsh J, Young JM, Harrison JD, Butow PN, Solomon MJ, Masya L, et al.

What is important in cancer care coordination? A qualitative investigation. European Journal of Cancer Care. 2011;**20**(2):220-227. DOI: 10.1111/j.1365-2354.2010.01187.x

[38] McAllister JW, Keehn RM, Rodgers R, Lock TM. Care coordination using a shared plan of care approach: From model to practice. Journal of Pediatric Nursing. 2018;**43**:88-96. DOI: 10.1016/j.pedn.2018.09.009

[39] Rotenstein L, Tucker S, Kakoza R, Tishler L, Zai A, Wu C. The critical components of an electronic care plan tool for primary care: An exploratory qualitative study. Journal of Innovation in Health Informatics. 2016;**23**(2):836. DOI: 10.14236/jhi.v23i2.836

[40] Porter ME. What is value in health care? The New England Journal of Medicine. 2010;**363**(26):2477-2481. DOI: 10.1056/NEJMp1011024

[41] Walradt J, Jackson HA. Adapting to the reimbursement landscape: The future of value-based care. Heart Failure Clinics. 2020;**16**(4):479-487. DOI: 10.1016/j.hfc.2020.06.008

[42] Henkel RJ, Maryland PA. The risks and rewards of value-based reimbursement. Frontiers of Health Services Management. 2015;**32**(2):3-16. Available from: https://pubmed.ncbi.nlm.nih.gov/26817266/

[43] Owolabi OR, Olatoye FO, Elufioye OA, Okunade B. Reviewing healthcare financial management: Strategies for cost-effective care. World Journal of Advanced Research and Reviews. 2024;**21**(2):958-966. DOI: 10.30574/wjarr.2024.21.2.0523

[44] Jawanjal RR. The influence of healthcare policies on hospital operations and management. International Journal of Research in Management. 2024;**6**(1):273-275. DOI: 10.33545/26648792.2024.v6.i1c.154

[45] Ibrahim AM, Abdel-Aziz HR, Mohamed HAH, Zaghamir DEF, Wahba NMI, Hassan GA, et al. Balancing confidentiality and care coordination: Challenges in patient privacy. BMC Nursing. 2024;**23**(1):564. DOI: 10.1186/s12912-024-02231-1

[46] Grabowski DC. Care coordination for dually eligible Medicare-Medicaid beneficiaries under the affordable care act. Journal of Aging & Social Policy. 2012;**24**(2):221-232. DOI: 10.1080/08959420.2012.659113

[47] Gluyas H. Patient-centred care: Improving healthcare outcomes. Nursing Standard. 2015;**30**(4):50-57. DOI: 10.7748/ns.30.4.50.e10186

[48] Dzau VJ, McClellan MB, McGinnis JM, Burke SP, Coye MJ, Diaz A, et al. Vital directions for health and health care: Priorities from a National Academy of Medicine Initiative. JAMA. 11 Apr 2017;**317**(14):1461-1470. DOI: 10.1001/jama.2017.1964

[49] Bao C, Bardhan IR. Performance of accountable care organizations: Health information technology and quality–efficiency trade-offs. Information Systems Research. Jun 2022;**33**(2):697-717. DOI: 10.1287/isre.2021.1080

[50] Zayas-Cabán T, Okubo TH, Posnack S. Priorities to accelerate workflow automation in health care. Journal of the American Medical Informatics Association. 2022;**30**(1):195-201. DOI: 10.1093/jamia/ocac197

[51] Turbow S, Hollberg JR, Ali MK. Electronic health record interoperability: How did we get here and how do we

move forward? JAMA Health Forum. 2021;**2**(3):e210253. DOI: 10.1001/jamahealthforum.2021.0253

[52] McMurray J, Hicks EM, Johnson H, Stolee P. 'Trying to find information is like hating yourself every day': The collision of electronic information systems in transition with patients in transition. Health Informatics Journal. 2013;**19**(3):218-232. DOI: 10.1177/1460458212467547

Section 6

Clinical Reasoning, Communication, and the Therapeutic Alliance

Chapter 8

Motivational Interview Applications for Aiding Therapeutic Alliance in the Era of Social Media Misinformation: An Integrative Review

Emmanuel Ohakpougwu and Craig Field

Abstract

The rise of social media as an important source of breaking news challenging traditional news outlets has also arguably given rise to an increase in misinformation. The explosion of this phenomenon during the COVID-19 pandemic led to its categorization as an "infodemic" by the WHO. Todays, healthcare provider cannot not overlook the influence misinformation on health topics can have on health behavior from medication adherence, lifestyle modification, to even acceptance of medical professional recommendation. Google Scholar, PubMed, Scopus, and Embase were the primary databases for literature search. "Motivational interview," "health misinformation," and "social media" were the search terms. After applying filters such as studies within the past 5 years, and screening for duplicates 44 articles were retained. This was pruned further by eliminating studies not directly addressing clinical application of motivational interview. Hence, 38 studies formed the core of this narrative review. About 36.8 (14) % were randomized controlled trials and experimentation, with 28.7 (4) % of the RCTs specifically examining the application of motivational interview in vaccine hesitancy which was the most for any field where RCTs were applied. Notably, 31.7 (12) % of all studies focused on motivational interview for vaccine hesitancy, indicating the prominence of this topic in the current research. Motivational interview application for vaccine hesitancy was the most discussed subject, which could be an indicator of the current climate in healthcare. There is an urgent need to diversify research on motivational interview across various health fields especially tackling health misinformation to help equip today's primary care providers.

Keywords: motivational interview, therapeutic alliance, social media, misinformation, health, patient

1. Introduction

1.1 Motivational interview origins and concept

Motivational interview (MI) is a process utilizing a conversational style to facilitate collaboration between the healthcare provider and patient in order to achieve a desired outcome [1]. Initially pioneered by William Miller in 1983 to help ensure behavioral changes in patients battling alcoholism, its application has expanded into other physical and mental healthcare contexts and has seen wide use in psychological research. Today, MI provides a non-confrontational and non-judgmental way to encourage behavioral change and strengthen the alliance between healthcare providers and patients. MI is rooted in the view that people have challenging behaviors, such as smoking, poor medication adherence, and insufficient exercise, and possess different levels of readiness to change such behavior [2]. Central to this concept is Janis and Mann's conflict theory of decision-making, which proposes that the advantages of healthy behaviors (e.g., better health outcomes) are almost always countered by the disadvantages of behavior change (e.g., significant effort). Hence, MI recognizes ambivalence as a key component of delay in poor behavior change rather than a lack of motivation, and if not identified and tackled, medical advice could be seen as an assault on freedom of choice, contributing to non-adherence or open disagreement [2]. Therefore, MI seeks to increase personal commitment to behavior change by intensifying personal reasons for behavior change in an empathy-abundant atmosphere [2]. There are four interview techniques in motivational interview, namely, the first to fifth intervention elements. The first intervention element emphasizes the use of open-ended questions in a bid to encourage confrontation of problem behavior, for example, "what worries you about your smoking" [2]. The second intervention element involves active listening to uncover and focus the patient's attention on their problem behavior. This gives room for self-exploration of the problem. The third element is affirmation, which has three arms: praise ("it is great that you want to handle your drinking"), recognition ("I can see that things are challenging for you"), and understanding ("It is clear to me that you are worried about the side effects of your medication"). The fourth element, summarizing, helps re-explore the contents of the patients' concerns that are significant driving forces for behavior change and re-echo them. The final intervention involves facilitating self-motivational statements, having created a cognizance of the dangers of poor behavior change, and then proceeding to concrete plans for behavior change. MI has been widely accepted as an evidence-based and effective method for promoting behavior change, treatment adherence, and sustaining therapeutic alliance between patient and health care provider [2]. Since its first design, MI has found greater application across other fields outside clinical psychology. For instance, studies have shown its effectiveness in helping post-acute coronary syndrome patients get motivated to begin cardiac rehabilitation, increase physical activity prescriptions by general practitioners upon agreement with patients, and also help in diabetes and weight management [3].

1.2 Medical misinformation and social media

Medical misinformation is information about medical issues presented as fact, but in reality, is false due to a lack of scientific evidence. However, this definition could also be extended to exaggeration of truths, misinterpretation, and wrong context applications [3]. Today, medical misinformation spans almost every topic in health care and has become so virulent that on most popular social media platforms, the top 1% of false news reached between 1000 and 100,000 people, as opposed to true facts, which barely got to 1000 people [4]. The ever-growing number of social media applications has led to increased democratization of access to, and production of information, occasionally called "creating content," leading to the virality of false claims. The COVID-19 pandemic exposed this challenge further, especially in the realm of health information, causing the WHO to rename this situation an infodemic where there is an explosion of false or misleading information in digital or physical environments, especially during a disease outbreak [5, 6]. A more positive attitude to alternative medicine, distrust in healthcare, less health literacy, racial/ethnic minority, higher religiosity, and older age have been shown to be positively correlated with increased susceptibility to health misinformation [7]. Studies have shown that 72% of people use the internet as the first source of health-related information and utilize web-based information to prepare for conversations with clinicians [7, 8]. Thus, health misinformation has real-life consequences, leading to delay in seeking medical care and expending resources on futile therapies, and sometimes death [9, 10]. Arguably, the most devastating consequence of health misinformation is that it erodes trust in medical science and breeds movements that might be anti-science, with real consequences for public health [11, 12]. Misinformation is hard to classify, and currently, 50 unique forms of misinformation have been identified, with fake news, manipulation, rumors, fabrication, and clickbait the most researched in literature [7, 13–15]. Understanding the mechanism by which social media supports the proliferation of misinformation is critical to any initiatives to tackle it in the clinic. Firstly, anecdotal evidence is at the heart of health disinformation, as we are drawn to stories of what people say has happened to them medically rather than statistical evidence [7]. Numerous studies have shown our inherent bias for anecdotal evidence, stories, over scientific evidence, especially when emotional engagement is high over a medical subject [16–19]. For instance, Parker Beck's improved autism symptoms after secretin injection during endoscopy became sensationalized, leading thousands of parents to require secretin injections for their children, and this demand resulted in 14 randomized controlled trials to disprove secretin as an effective treatment for autism [20]. Beyond anecdotal evidence, health misinformation is enhanced by echo chambers and algorithms because they bar people from exposure to differing views besides theirs, thereby reinforcing tightly held ideas [21]. Studies have shown that more than 50% of blog readers search for blogs supporting their own views [21, 22]. To make matters worse, prior exposure to misinformation increased one's capacity to promote misinformation by over 18%, with a 91% likelihood to spread misinformed headlines despite knowing they were false [23, 24]. As dissatisfaction with Western medicine has grown, the doctor-patient relationship has soured, and belief in alternative medicine or therapies has soared. In fact, the misinformation about alternative therapies is so pervasive that one study found that out of the first 50 websites when one googled "weight loss," 47 focused on slimming aids and dietary supplements without any evidence [25]. It is worth noting that evidence demonstrating how pharmaceutical marketing influences physician prescription also impact doctor-patient relationship negatively. This serves to make the clinical encounter golden opportunity to address a lot of patient concerns and effectively make patients advocates for the positive reputation health care providers [26–29]. Hence, in this paper, we aim to explore the current state of research in motivational interview for combating health misinformation and explore avenues for improvement in the clinical setting.

1.3 Evidence for motivational interview effectiveness across clinical contexts

Recent meta-analyses and randomized controlled trials (RCTs) demonstrate the effectiveness of motivational interview (MI) as a clinical intervention across various health contexts. Specifically, a robust meta-analysis by Lundahl et al. highlighted MI's efficacy in improving health-related behaviors, such as substance use reduction and weight management [30]. The study aggregated results from numerous trials, illustrating that MI has consistently led to meaningful improvements in patient outcomes [30]. Further, research by Heckman et al. focused specifically on smoking cessation, reporting significant positive effects when MI was employed, thereby reinforcing its application in tobacco dependency contexts [31].

An important systematic review by Barnes and Ivezaj examined MI's applicability in primary care settings for weight loss, revealing that MI significantly aids in patient compliance and effectively addresses the unique barriers often present in such environments [32]. Similarly, the study by Cascaes et al. demonstrated MI's effectiveness in enhancing oral health interventions aimed at preventing dental caries, indicating MI's broad applicability in promoting health behaviors beyond behavioral health settings [33]. These studies converge on the point that MI's adaptability to diverse clinical situations provides a compelling case for its implementation in addressing health-related challenges.

1.4 Theoretical foundations of MI beyond conflict theory

The theoretical underpinnings of motivational interview extend beyond conflict theory, integrating perspectives from various psychological and behavioral models. Central to MI's approach are the constructs of the Transtheoretical Model (TTM) and Self-Determination Theory (SDT). The TTM outlines stages of change that individuals progress through when modifying behavior, aligning seamlessly with MI's intent to support individuals in exploring their ambivalence and readiness for change [34]. This model emphasizes the tailored conversations that MI fosters, allowing practitioners to meet clients at their current stage of motivation.

Self-determination theory complements the foundations of MI by focusing on intrinsic motivation and the psychological needs for autonomy and competence. A motivational interview framework aligns with SDT principles, fostering an environment in which clients feel empowered to change through supportive communication [35]. By aligning with autonomy, MI encourages individuals to own their decisions, thus enhancing commitment to change.

1.5 Mechanisms of misinformation propagation

Understanding how misinformation propagates involves insights from cognitive psychology, behavioral economics, and elements of algorithmic bias inherent in digital communication platforms. Cognitive psychology elucidates how individuals often resort to cognitive biases when absorbing and interpreting health information, leading to the reinforcement of misinformation beliefs [36]. The human tendency to favor information that confirms existing beliefs (confirmation bias) is a critical mechanism driving misinformation spread, particularly in health contexts where personal beliefs override factual correctness.

Behavioral economics adds another layer by illustrating how decision-making processes are influenced by context and framing effects. Individuals may be swayed toward certain health choices by the manner in which information is presented; for instance, loss aversion can compel individuals to overestimate the risks associated with health interventions [37]. The interplay of these mechanisms is compounded by algorithmic biases on social media platforms, which often promote sensationalized misinformation over factual content to maximize engagement and visibility [38]. Understanding these dynamics is crucial for developing effective strategies within motivational interview to counter misinformation by guiding individuals toward a more informed and critical engagement with health information.

2. Methodology

A literature review was conducted using Google Scholar, PubMed, Scopus, and Embase, focusing on the keywords "motivational interview," "health misinformation," "health communication," and "social media." The initial search included poring over 100 pages of Google Scholar. After applying filters for relevance, recency, and duplicates, 44 articles remained. Further screening based on direct relevance (studies focusing on the application of MI in the clinical setting) reduced this number to 38 studies, which formed the basis of the review.

Inclusion criteria: Studies conducted globally, regardless of language, studies in a clinical setting, or geared toward in-person/telehealth settings for motivational interview. Studies published from 2020 to 2025. Studies without a paywall.

Exclusion criteria: After full text screenings, articles not addressing at least two key terms/concepts simultaneously, such as social media use, health communication, misinformation, and motivational interview, were removed from this review. Studies older than 5 years, as well as studies with a paywall, were excluded (**Table 1**).

3. Results

Among the selected studies, 36.8 (14) % were randomized controlled trials and experimentation, with 28.7 (4) % of the RCTs specifically examining the application of motivational interview in vaccine hesitancy, which was the most for any field where RCTs were applied. Notably, 31.7 (12) % of all studies focused on motivational interview for vaccine hesitancy, indicating the prominence of this topic in current research. This is in line with the explosion of research in this area following the COVID-19 pandemic and attendant high levels of misinformation.

3.1 Efficacy of MI

A meta-analysis concluded that the effect of motivational interview on health behavior was significant, with an odds ratio of 1.55 as opposed to standard treatment or no treatment [51]. This study demonstrated that MI was most effective in the following areas: substance use, improving physical activity, dental hygiene, body weight, and treatment adherence [51]. An RCT conducted for 1 year showed that brief-MI by dentists gave room for patients to discuss several health concerns beyond their traditional appointments, such as nutrition, mental health, and lifestyle modification [52]. However, a single study negated these results, and this systematic review reported that MI showed no positive effects on medication adherence for people with stroke and transient ischemic attack [71]. Another systematic review of randomized

Title of paper	Type of study	Summary of motivational interview application	Health field discussed
Vaccine hesitancy educational tools for healthcare providers and trainees: A scoping review	Scoping review	Interventions for knowledge sharing and communication training focused on health care providers. Interventions focused only on doctors, and no studies explored emotion management for difficult conversations.	Vaccines/vaccine hesitancy [39]
Interrogating the pill: Rising distrust and the reshaping of health risk perceptions in the social media age	Qualitative study: An exploratory online observation and an in-depth interview study with 19 informants in Germany and Denmark	Social media was found to play a central role in how young women perceived the risk and safety of contraceptives. Consequently, this has led to the delegitimizing of gynecologists and led to the rise of peer influencers.	Contraceptives and gynecological care [40]
What works to increase vaccination uptake	Narrative review	Reviews how the Increasing Vaccination Model works. Health provider recommendation is the most potent factor in increased vaccine uptake, but it is not clear why and how this works.	Vaccination [41]
Communicating with vaccine-hesitant parents	Narrative review	A presumptive format to initiate vaccine conversation, this approach presumes parents will vaccinate and frames vaccination as a default behavior. Furthermore, motivational interview and tailoring messages to increase salience led to positive outcomes.	Vaccination [42]
Refuting spurious COVID-19 treatment claims reduces demand and misinformation sharing	Quantitative: experiment	Enhanced and tentative refutation of misinformation led to reduced demand for misinformation as well as its promotion by 29 and 55%, respectively. Refutations based on evidence-based guidelines founded on psychological research are more effective for managing misinformation than tentative refutations employed by health authorities.	Effect of Vitamin E on COVID-19 [23]

Title of paper	Type of study	Summary of motivational interview application	Health field discussed
Motivational interview from the pediatricians' perspective: assessments after a 2-day training for physicians caring for adolescents with chronic medical conditions (CMCs)	Mixed methods	This study evaluated the experiences of pediatricians with a 2-day motivational interview (MI) course, finding it valuable for working with adolescents with chronic medical conditions, but highlighting challenges such as short training duration and lack of time, and recommending booster sessions for sustained effectiveness. • Pediatricians found motivational interview (MI) to be a valuable tool for working with adolescents with chronic medical conditions (CMCs), with 95% considering it necessary for their clinical work. • A 2-day MI course was effective in improving communication behavior, but challenges such as short training duration and lack of time were identified. • Comprehensive integration of MI into clinical routine is challenging due to practical constraints, despite its perceived benefits in strengthening physician-patient connections.	Pediatrics [43]
Fidelity of a motivational interview intervention for improving return to work for people with musculoskeletal disorders	Randomized controlled trial	The study evaluated the fidelity of a motivational interview intervention delivered by social insurance caseworkers to improve return to work for individuals with musculoskeletal disorders, finding that most caseworkers did not reach proficiency levels despite thorough training and supervision, indicating a need for extensive practice and support to master motivational interview.	Musculoskeletal disorders [44]
The impact of a syndemic theory-based intervention on HIV transmission risk behavior among men who have sex with men in India: Pretest-posttest non-equivalent comparison group trial	Controlled intervention study	Syndemic theory guided motivational interview-based HIV intervention among men having sex with men increased consistent condom use by 16.4% and led to a significant reduction in problematic alcohol use and depression. Mediation analyses indicated that improvements in condom use self-efficacy contributed to the intervention's effectiveness.	HIV [45]

Title of paper	Type of study	Summary of motivational interview application	Health field discussed
Music therapy combined with motivational interview	Randomized controlled trial	Music therapy combined with motivational interview on young and middle-aged patients with anxiety and depression after percutaneous coronary intervention (PCI) for myocardial infarction (MI), finding that this combined intervention can effectively regulate mood, reduce anxiety and depression symptoms, and stimulate healthy behavioral habits.	Mental health and cardiology [46]
Fake news and science denier attacks on vaccines. What can you do?	Opinion piece	• Misinformation about vaccines spreads rapidly and has serious consequences on health decisions and trust in immunization advice. • Five tactics used by vaccine deniers include conspiracy, fake experts, selectivity, impossible expectations, and misrepresentation and false logic. • Healthcare providers are cautioned against myth-busting and knowledge-dumping as these have been shown to have no real positive influence on vaccination.	Vaccination [47]
Importance of lifestyle modification on cardiovascular risk reduction counseling strategies to maximize patient outcomes	Commentary	The paper emphasizes the importance of lifestyle modification in reducing cardiovascular risk, highlighting the need for healthcare providers to assess patient readiness to change and use strategies like motivational interview to facilitate behavior change, with a focus on addressing foundational risk factors and combining lifestyle modifications with cardioprotective medications. • Lifestyle modification and behavior change can slow or reverse the progression of atherosclerotic coronary heart disease (CHD). • Modifying unhealthy behaviors is a significant opportunity to improve health and reduce premature death, accounting for approximately 40% of all deaths in the United States. • Brief lifestyle counseling by allied health professionals can be highly effective in achieving favorable patient outcomes.	Cardio-rehabilitation [48]

Title of paper	Type of study	Summary of motivational interview application	Health field discussed
The empathetic refutational interview to tackle vaccine misconceptions: Four randomized experiments	Randomized experiment	The paper introduces and tests the "Empathetic Refutational Interview" (ERI), a novel multicomponent intervention for healthcare professionals to address anti-vaccination misconceptions while maintaining empathy. Empathetic Refutational Interview (ERI) produced small effects on increasing vaccine acceptance and lowering support for anti-vaccination arguments compared to control conditions. • Affirming participants' concerns significantly increased support for refutations and subsequent information, with large effects compared to controls. • Tailored refutations were more compelling and increased trust and openness toward healthcare professionals, indicating the importance of empathy in communication.	Vaccine [49]
The experience of health professionals with misinformation and its impact on their job practice: Qualitative interview study	Qualitative study	Health professionals view misinformation differently depending on the context and are developing pathways to address it through education and communication. • Lack of trust in health professionals is attributed to factors like alternative information sources, doubts about experience, and limited time for patient interaction. • Main recommendations include listening to patients, allocating more time, and using evidence-based resources to build trust and combat misinformation.	Primary care [50]
The influence of patient-centered communication on psychological distress: The chain mediating role of health-related self-efficacy and healthy lifestyle behaviors, and the moderating role of social media use	Retrospective study	This study found that patient-centered communication is negatively associated with psychological distress, with health-related self-efficacy and healthy lifestyle behaviors playing a chain mediating role, and social media use enhancing the positive impact on health-related self-efficacy.	Primary care [51]

Title of paper	Type of study	Summary of motivational interview application	Health field discussed
Communication pathways from the emergency department to community mental health services: A systematic review	Systematic review	This systematic review synthesizes evidence on strategies to enhance communication pathways between emergency departments and community mental health services, identifying support coordination, motivational interview, electronic record enhancement, and phone follow-up as effective in improving continuity of care and reducing re-presentations. Support coordination, motivational interview, education, and enhanced electronic records can improve continuity of care and reduce ED re-presentations for mental health concerns.	Emergency medicine care and mental health care [52]
Motivational interview: An evidence-based approach for use in medical practice	Meta-analyses	• Motivational interview (MI) has statistically significant effects on various health behaviors compared to standard treatment or no treatment, with an odds ratio of 1.55. • Significant effects are noted in substance consumption, physical activity, dental hygiene, body weight, treatment adherence, and mortality. • MI is useful for strengthening motivation for behavioral change and promoting treatment adherence.	Primary care [2]
Hot topics emerged from a brief motivational interview: A randomized controlled trial	Randomized controlled trial	The study aimed to analyze health topics emerging from brief motivational interview (MI) compared to traditional oral hygiene instructions (OHI). Fifty-eight periodontal maintenance patients were randomized to brief-MI or traditional OHI for a 1-year clinical trial, with audio recordings transcribed and coded. Brief-MI evoked more topics toward total health, with increased discussion of oral home care, oral diseases, lifestyle, nutrition, emotional/mental health, and general health compared to traditional OHI.	Dental care [53]

Title of paper	Type of study	Summary of motivational interview application	Health field discussed
Addressing parental vaccine hesitancy toward childhood vaccines in the United States: A systematic literature review of communication interventions and strategies	Systematic literature review	Interventions should target parents early in pregnancy, tailor information to the audience, and present vaccination as the default approach. Effective interventions incorporate dialog, balanced information, storytelling with gists, and carefully chosen messengers like healthcare providers. Technology should be used cautiously to promote vaccination, addressing misinformation and improving vaccine literacy and critical thinking skills.	Vaccine [54]
Counselors' verbal behaviors and skills that elicit participants' change or sustain talk in virtual motivational interview for physical activity among older adults	Qualitative study	This study examines the influence of counselors' verbal behaviors on participants' change talk and sustain talk during virtual motivational interview for physical activity among older adults, finding that MI-consistent behaviors elicit change talk, sustain talk, and follow/neutral talk, while MI-inconsistent behaviors and "other" behaviors also elicit change talk, providing insights into how MI works in virtual settings.	Physical activity and geriatrics [55]
Culturally-based challenges to and recommendations for delivering adherence counseling in a multicultural biomedical HIV prevention trial in four African countries	Mixed methods study integrated into a clinical trial for open-label dapivirine ring.	The paper examines the challenges and recommendations for delivering adherence counseling in a multicultural biomedical HIV prevention trial, highlighting the importance of flexibility and community involvement in adapting interventions to address cultural barriers. Counselors encountered barriers such as participants struggling with culturally incongruent pictorial guides and partner disapproval. • The intervention's flexibility allowed counselors to adapt language and examples, which was seen as an asset in overcoming cultural barriers. • Despite challenges, participant comprehension and receptiveness to Options Counseling were reported as high.	HIV [56]

Title of paper	Type of study	Summary of motivational interview application	Health field discussed
Tiered clinician vaccine communication strategy to improve childhood vaccine uptake: A cluster randomized clinical trial	Cluster randomized clinical trial	In a cluster randomized clinical trial involving 937 parent-child dyads at 24 clinics in Washington and Colorado, a tiered clinician vaccine communication strategy did not significantly improve vaccine uptake among children of parents with negative vaccine attitudes overall, although it showed increased odds of timely vaccination in Washington State.	Vaccination [57]
The potential influence of depressive symptoms on outcomes from a brief motivational intervention in patients referred to cardiac rehabilitation	Randomized clinical trial	A brief motivational intervention improves cardiac rehabilitation participation outcomes regardless of depressive symptoms, although socioeconomic factors may influence perceived suitability, and the intervention is perceived favorably by patients across different levels of depressive symptoms.	Mental health and cardiology [58]
Efficacy of behavioral activation in the treatment of negative symptoms in people with schizophrenia spectrum disorders: A systematic review	Systematic review	This systematic review of two studies suggests that behavioral activation may hold potential as an alternative treatment for negative symptoms in individuals with schizophrenia spectrum disorders, despite limited and low-quality evidence, and highlights its simplicity and adaptability for broader accessibility.	Mental health [59]
Comparative effectiveness of parent-based interventions to support injured children	Randomized clinical trial	A comparative effectiveness trial found that both Link for Injured Kids and Trauma Education were effective in reducing posttraumatic stress, depression, and improving quality of life in hospitalized injured children, with Link showing additional benefits in improving emotional and behavioral outcomes, particularly in rural settings. The Link Program taught parents motivational interview and stress screening skills. Both Link and Trauma Education interventions were associated with similar improvements in posttraumatic stress symptoms, depression, and quality of life in hospitalized injured children. • The Link intervention showed notable improvements in child emotional behaviors and mild improvements in conduct and peer behaviors.	Pediatrics, Emergency Medicine [60]

Title of paper	Type of study	Summary of motivational interview application	Health field discussed
Effect of a transtheoretical model-based intervention and motivational interview on hyperphosphatemia management *via* telehealth (TMT program) among hemodialysis patients during the COVID-19 pandemic	Randomized controlled trial	The study found that a transtheoretical model-based intervention combined with motivational interview, delivered *via* telehealth, significantly reduced serum phosphorus levels and improved dietary consumption behavior, self-efficacy, and adherence to phosphate binders among hemodialysis patients during the COVID-19 pandemic.	Nephrology [61]
Effectiveness of a training program for the management of risky alcohol use in primary care professionals based on motivational interview	Randomized open-label controlled clinical trial	The study demonstrates the effectiveness of a training program for primary care professionals in increasing knowledge and skills for managing patients with risky alcohol use and improving motivational interview skills. • The training program was effective in improving the knowledge of primary care professionals about managing risky alcohol use. • There was a significant improvement in motivational interview skills among the professionals who received the training. • The training program was effective in increasing knowledge and skills to manage patients with risky excessive alcohol consumption.	Substance use [62]
The feasibility of motivational interview on adherence to care practices, emotional intelligence, and dispositional optimism among patients with permanent pacemakers	Randomized controlled trial	The study concluded that motivational interview (MI) improves patient adherence to care practices for those with permanent pacemakers. MI fosters emotional intelligence (EI) and optimism among patients post-implantation. Statistically significant improvements in self-care adherence and EI were observed after MI implementation. The findings support MI as a feasible approach for enhancing patient outcomes in this population.	MI for cardiac rehabilitation after insertion of a pacemaker [63]

Title of paper	Type of study	Summary of motivational interview application	Health field discussed
Effectiveness of the transtheoretical model-based motivational interview on glycaemic control among adults with Type 2 diabetes: A systematic review and meta-analysis of randomized control trials	Systematic review and meta-analysis	The meta-analysis supports the effectiveness of the TTM-based MI intervention for improving self-management behaviors in T2D patients. It emphasizes better glycemic control as a significant outcome of the intervention. The findings suggest that tailored strategies can facilitate behavior change in T2D patients. The paper calls for further rigorous trials due to the moderate to high risk of bias in included studies.	Endocrinology [64]
Predictors of COVID-19 vaccine acceptance and hesitancy among healthcare workers in Southern California: Not just "anti" vs. "pro" vaccine	Cross-sectional survey	The study evaluates COVID-19 vaccination attitudes among healthcare workers in Southern California, highlighting diverse vaccine hesitancy categories. It emphasizes the need for targeted interventions to increase vaccine confidence among healthcare workers. The paper discusses the importance of addressing the root causes of vaccine hesitancy, regardless of governmental mandates. It suggests using behavioral economics and prosocial messaging to enhance vaccination intentions in hesitant groups. The research indicates that political affiliation, education, and income significantly influence vaccination status.	Vaccination hesitancy [65]
A field test of empathetic refutational and motivational interview to address vaccine hesitancy among patients	Mixed methods field test	The study observed larger improvements in attitudes toward vaccines in MI and ERI groups compared to the control group. Physicians expressed discomfort in interactions with patients holding anti-vaccination beliefs. The findings suggest that motivational interview can enhance physician-patient communication. Participants indicated a desire for more effective discussions about vaccination. The ERI framework is introduced, featuring a 4-step structure for patient interaction. Key steps include eliciting concerns, providing information, and addressing misconceptions.	Primary care [66]

Title of paper	Type of study	Summary of motivational interview application	Health field discussed
Effectiveness of group and individual counseling interventions on COVID-19 vaccination intention among industrial employees in Romania	Intervention study	The study identified key factors contributing to vaccine hesitancy, including age, education, marital status, and chronic diseases. Both group and individual counseling interventions significantly increased vaccine willingness among participants. The research highlights the role of trusted healthcare professionals in promoting vaccine acceptance through tailored communication strategies.	Vaccination [67]
Optimizing education to improve COVID-19 vaccination rates in a federally qualified health center	Quality improvement project	COVID-19 vaccination hesitancy is prevalent in underserved communities, and education can combat this issue. Documentation of vaccine status increased vaccination rates significantly after interventions. Physician confidence in discussing COVID-19 vaccines improved from 2.8 to 4.3 out of 5. Misinformation about COVID-19 vaccines was widespread, impacting patient education.	Vaccination [68]
Increasing COVID-19 vaccination rates among patients with serious mental illness: A pilot intervention study	Pilot intervention study	Incorporating vaccination discussions in psychiatric visits can enhance vaccination rates among patients with serious mental illness. Psychiatric providers can effectively address vaccine hesitancy and provide accurate information. Strategies to ensure completed vaccination series should involve family and care teams. Allowing vaccinations at mental health practices would improve accessibility. Expanding psychiatrists' roles in preventive care can protect marginalized patients.	Vaccination in psychiatry [69]

Title of paper	Type of study	Summary of motivational interview application	Health field discussed
The impact of pharmacy care and motivational interview on improving medication adherence in patients with cardiovascular diseases: A systematic review of randomized controlled trials	Systematic review	The review indicates that motivational interview may enhance medication adherence in patients with cardiovascular disease (CVD). Evidence suggests further research is needed to explore the impact of motivational interview on clinical outcomes. The findings highlight the potential of motivational interview as a strategy in pharmacy practice.	Medication adherence and pharmacy practice [70]
Effectiveness of motivational interview on medication adherence for the prevention of recurrent stroke or transient ischemic attack: Systematic review of randomized controlled trials	Systematic review	The evidence on motivational interview (MI) is inconclusive for improving medication adherence to prevent recurrent stroke and TIA. No significant differences were found in quality of life (QoL) or clinical outcomes related to MI. There is a need for well-designed studies and evaluations of MI as a complex intervention for stroke patients.	Medication adherence and stroke [71]
Effectiveness of motivational interview in smoking groups in primary healthcare: A community-based randomized cluster trial	Cluster randomized controlled trial	The study found that motivational interview combined with cognitive behavioral therapy (CBT) was effective for smoking cessation in groups. The smoking cessation rate was 61.8% in the motivational interview group compared to 47.7% in the control group. The mean session attendance was slightly higher in the motivational interview group (3.1) than in the control group. The completion rate was 65.2% for the motivational interview group and 57.6% for the control group.	Mental health [72]

Table 1.
Studies on motivational interview across different health contexts.

controlled trials reported that pharmacist-led MI was effective in ensuring medication adherence in patients with cardiovascular disease broadly [70].

3.2 MI and vaccine hesitancy

Almost no field of medicine is safe from the onslaught of medical misinformation because of social media use. From rising concerns about contraceptive use across Germany and Denmark, to childhood vaccinations [39, 40]. Handling vaccine hesitancy was repeatedly deemed to be the most difficult for health workers, and various studies advocated for health workers to avoid myth-busting when caring for adults who are against vaccination [40]. A systematic literature review showed that balanced interventions incorporating dialog, storytelling, and balancing information while being cautious about the use of technology in promoting vaccination were the most impactful for managing vaccine hesitancy [2]. Overall, most papers shared that healthcare worker recommendations were often the most potent factor in vaccine uptake and often worked when motivational interview pertaining to vaccine messages were tailored [41, 42]. On the other hand, a cross-sectional survey showed that healthcare providers could also express vaccine hesitancy, which can be damaging to public health [65]. And designing MI to target this group is also important. MI was also shown to be a valuable tool for tackling vaccines in psychiatric patients, especially when offered *via* coordination of family and care teams [69].

3.3 Clinical approach to MI

On combating health disinformation in the clinic, two papers disagreed. A study exploring the outcomes of health workers refuting claims that Vitamin E prevents COVID-19 found that refuting health misinformation using evidence-based guidelines led to 29% less demand for more misinformation and a 55% reduction in the health misinformation promotion [23]. On the other hand, another study found myth-busting/refutation was seen as a poor approach with little to no effects in improving vaccine uptake, for instance [47]. However, a field test showed that empathetic refutational interviews worked best as this created a conducive environment for clinicians to talk about vaccine hesitancy and made patients interested in further conversations [66]. Furthermore, a randomized experiment using empathetic refutational interviewing reported small positive effects on vaccine acceptance; nevertheless, affirming patients' concerns made them more amenable to refutations [49]. Furthermore, a cluster randomized trial demonstrated that motivational interview could fail when negative attitudes are strongly held, as seen in a tiered vaccine communication strategy led by clinicians [55]. Nevertheless, this study showed that even if parents might disagree strongly on certain aspects of vaccination, they might still ensure that vaccination is timely for their children while still interrogating their beliefs. Thus, MI might not lead to immediate verbal agreement or change in tightly held beliefs but could produce change as recipients reflect subsequently. The trans-theoretical model for MI was shown to be superior in helping patients with type 2 diabetes, leading to reduced glycaemic levels and better self-management [64].

3.4 Constraints to using MI and secondary effects

A physician-led motivational interview was at the epicenter of most studies. A mixed methods study which evaluated the experiences of pediatricians using a 2-day course of MI showed that they found it particularly useful for discussing chronic medical conditions with adolescents, with 95% considering it necessary for their clinical work [43]. However, time constraints in its application in the clinic were significant concerns [48]. Beyond clinical constraints, there are concerns about reaching proficiency in MI among users and the impact of the short duration of training. This was witnessed not only in clinical staff but also among social workers in an RCT who never reached proficiency in MI during the study, indicating a need for extensive training and possible refreshers [44]. Several studies showed that motivational interview could have downstream effects in a targeted intervention, which can improve overall health outcomes [45, 46]. For instance, a motivational interview-based intervention for HIV led to a 16% increase in condom use in men having sex with men but also had downstream effects such as a reduction in substance use and depression [45]. This demonstrates the value of motivational interview in single-session intervention/ brief interventions and is supported by its value in helping initiate lifestyle modifications for patients at risk of cardiovascular disease [48].

3.5 MI in telehealth

A retrospective study concluded that in the presence of patient-centered communication, social media use was in fact a positive influence leading to improved self-management [49]. Only two studies explored the role of MI in a virtual setting, for example, in telehealth. A qualitative study showed that counselors applying the principles of MI appropriately with older adults about physical activity led to participants getting to the stages of sustain talk and follow-up, where they were ready to implement healthy behavior [2]. Also, an RCT employing the transtheoretical model-based motivational interview *via* tele-health showed that MI reduced serum phosphorus levels due to adherence to treatment with phosphate binders and dietary consumption among patients on hemodialysis [60].

3.6 MI in mental health

Beyond substance use, motivational interview was shown to have applications in reducing the prevalence of posttraumatic stress and depression among injured children who were hospitalized and their parents alike [59]. Also, a systematic review showed that it was an important adjunct to behavioral activation in treating negative symptoms in individuals with schizophrenia spectrum disorders [57]. In a cluster randomized trial, MI was shown to reduce smoking by over 60% when applied alongside cognitive behavioral therapy, as opposed to cognitive behavioral therapy being the sole form of treatment [72].

4. Discussion

Vaccine hesitancy, the delay in acceptance or refusal of safe vaccines despite their availability [59, 73], which has become a widespread challenge, especially post-COVID-19, featured prominently in most studies, indicating congruence with the times. The drivers of vaccine hesitancy are multifactorial and may even depend on the specific vaccine being considered, but all studies in this review focused on "patient-centered" factors such as mistrust in medical institutions. Even though clinicians showed an eagerness to handle misinformation about vaccines, several factors were identified as constraints: time to carry out motivational interview as well as training for motivational interview [43, 48, 74]. Considering these factors, MI may well fail as a tool in the clinical setting for combating health misinformation, not because of inefficacy but due to provider constraints. In fact, one study showed healthcare providers never reached proficiency in its use [44]. Hence, there is a key need to understand how various strategies for handling vaccine misinformation are incorporated into MI during a clinic visit. One school of thought actively advocates against myth-busting, citing the absence of behavior change and demonstrating that it might rather serve to make parents entrenched in their position [40]. We argue that this approach might be too pessimistic, and a rather balanced approach, applying methods such as empathy, storytelling, and open dialog, might give more room for behavior change [2]. In having a constructive discussion about vaccines with hesitant parents, the healthcare provider's approach should go beyond showing evidence of solid science for vaccine safety, but also applying a deep knowledge of psychological reactance and deliberate enhancement of patients' science media literacy to combat it [75]. Psychological reactance is an emotionally charged defensive response when there is a perceived threat to one's freedom [56, 76]. Hence, healthcare providers must avoid binary questions such as, "are you worried about the vaccine"? to "what have you heard about the vaccine that worries you" [63]. These questions enable patients to engage fully in their concerns from side effects, vaccine development process, or information on social media, and gain insights to re-evaluate their position on vaccines [60, 77]. Validating the patient's concerns comes next, and this effectively demonstrates empathy, reduced defensiveness, and prepares the patient to engage further. Also, by focusing on the patients' positive intentions, an atmosphere for constructive collaborative engagement emerges [64].

Another prominent recurring theme is MI use in medication adherence, especially for chronic illness. Medication non-adherence is a real challenge to the prognosis of many medical conditions, and at least 50% of the time, patients fail to adhere to their medication regimen [19, 78–80]. Medication non-adherence is multifactorial, ranging from lack of access to medications to intentional action not to take medications. Generally, MI was viewed as reliable for managing chronic diseases in patients with chronic kidney disease, being consistent with diet recommendations while on dialysis, to older adults with comorbid conditions, maintaining physical exercise [81]. However, no studies in this review evaluated patients for up to 24 months or longer to ascertain if new behaviors from medication adherence to physical exercise were adhered to. In the presence of medication fatigue, this opens a new challenge for using MI. When the benefits of medication adherence are tied to the prevention of future illness, there can be reluctance to continue treatment [82]. The need for chronic daily medicine is often lost on patients as missing doses does not have an immediate consequence, and the fear of becoming dependent on medication hangs over treatment. Finally, depression among patients with chronic illness is also a core reason for poor medication adherence, as patients with depression are three times more likely to skip medications [83]. In patients with diabetes, for instance, depression has been implicated as a key reason for poor medication adherence, physical inactivity, poor glycaemic control, and disability [19]. For hypertension and diabetes, it has been shown that even basic education and understanding about the ills of the condition still do not reflect an improvement in medication adherence [84]. In fact, a cluster randomized control trial showed that the effect of MI wanes within a 6-to-12-month period from initiation [85]. These warrants adjusting health care provider expectations as well as further training in managing "relapses" or negative changes in behavior. Furthermore, as health care provider support remains consistent, then a patient's sense of self-efficacy will become enhanced, enabling them to take control of their blood pressure management, leading to overall well-being long-term [86]. In the same vein, MI has been shown to be successful in promoting healthy eating behavior [87, 88]. The concept of secondary or downstream effects of MI is an important reason to continue MI in the face of obvious behavior change. For instance, tackling substance use among men having sex with men amounted to increased use of condoms, which was the primary behavior change being studied [45]. Since other factors, such as depression and "treatment fatigue," might influence medication and physical activity adherence, MI could potentially lead to a resolution of those concerns, thus helping achieve positive behavior change.

In this review, MI was shown to have applications in mental health care beyond its use in addiction. Its efficacy was ascertained in managing symptoms of depression, and PTSD [89] was similar to other studies demonstrating similar effects in patients with anxiety disorders from OCD, GAD, to PTSD, leading to increased treatment seeking, especially in those not already seeking care, as well as treatment attendance [90–93]. In patients with depression, MI has also been noted to be useful both for supporting entry into care for depression, managing suicidal ideation, and adherence to antidepressants [94]. In severe mental illness, MI served as an adjunct to behavior activation, helping to manage negative symptoms and comorbid conditions such as substance use, and this is corroborated by research proving that a single session of MI led to greater hospital review and reduced tobacco use in patients diagnosed with schizoaffective disorder when compared to those receiving only psychological counseling [95]. Also, a combination of MI and CBT has been shown to increase antipsychotic adherence and positive attitudes toward treatment 18 months post discharge in patients with schizophrenia [96, 97]. For young people dealing with cannabis, alcohol, and cigarette use, a single-session motivational interview was enough to cause a significant reduction in drug use at follow-up 3 months later [98] and serves as an essential addition to the first session of psychotherapy [99]. Thus, MI can be applied in underserved areas where there is a shortage of the mental healthcare workforce.

The heterogeneity in the implementation of MI across various settings and studies also affects interpretations of its effectiveness. Additionally, the intervention's effectiveness is intricately linked to the clinician's level of competency in MI and the contextual nuances of the patient population engaged during interventions [36, 46, 100]. Furthermore, the scarcity of longitudinal studies evaluating the long-term impacts of motivational interview on patient attitudes toward misinformation in various health contexts is a critical research gap. While the existing literature highlights the importance of healthcare professionals in curbing misinformation, studies focusing on patient-centered approaches using MI to address misinformation directly remain underexplored [101]. Also, there is a need to advance research on motivational interview beyond vaccine hesitancy to other issues such as diet and medication. Integrating MI with larger public health frameworks is also an under-researched aspect. The research articles in this review overly focus on MI application in vaccine hesitancy tied to the COVID-19 vaccine, but there might be certain nuances peculiar to hesitancy to the Hepatitis B vaccine that have been missed as a result.

5. Conclusion

MI has an important role to play in today's healthcare ecosystem, especially with increasing distrust of healthcare workers across various sectors. Providing MI in a clinical setting affords the clinician room to address misinformation about health spread on social media and help steer patients toward adopting evidence-based care and healthy behaviors. Nevertheless, the efficacy of MI might be limited by provider training in its application and the time allotted to clinical reviews. Hence, healthcare institutions must make an effort to invest in extensive training and refresher courses for healthcare providers to ensure that their skills in MI are up to date. Furthermore, training in tailoring MI to specific scenarios is of utmost importance. This will enable clinicians to tackle the time constraints in high-volume clinical settings and increase the efficacy of MI for underserved populations. Digitizing MI might offer an avenue to ensure that positive behavior change does not wane over months. Debunking myths held by patients head-on is shown to increase resistance, but open dialog and empathetic refuting provide the clinician the opportunity to tackle misinformation and enable patients to begin the road to behavior change, albeit these efforts might not yield fruit in the interim. This is especially crucial when managing patients with chronic medical conditions who might develop fatigue with following medical advice. Utilizing MI might address secondary causes of a possible medication non-adherence, for instance, such as depression, and in turn, consequently lead to the expected behavior change.

Doctors remain the focus of studies on MI implementation; however, the current landscape would benefit from studying MI training and application for other staff, such as pharmacists and nurses, especially in underserved areas, when the former might not be available. This is also important to avoid contradictory approaches in managing patient concerns, which can only serve to deepen medical distrust. There is an urgent need for long-term studies exploring MI use in the health misconceptions shared by patients to ascertain if changes in beliefs and behavior were sustained over time or if patients resorted to their old beliefs reinforced by social media. There is a notable absence of research that intricately reconciles motivational interview techniques with comprehensive strategies designed to counteract misinformation propagation. While existing literature establishes MI's effectiveness in motivating individuals toward healthy behaviors, it does not adequately explore integrated frameworks that concurrently address misinformation in the health communication landscape.

Author details

Emmanuel Ohakpougwu[1*] and Craig Field[2]

1 School of Health Sciences Research, Chiang Mai University, Thailand

2 Bantuk Recovery and Rehabilitation Center, Accra, Ghana

*Address all correspondence to: emmanuelebuka828@gmail.com

References

[1] Emery RL, Wimmer M. Motivational interview. In: StatPearls [Internet]. Treasure Island (FL): StatPearls Publishing; 2025. Available from: https://www.ncbi.nlm.nih.gov/books/NBK589705/#_article-148671_s2_

[2] Bischof G, Bischof A, Rumpf HJ. Motivational interview: An evidence-based approach for use in medical practice. Deutsches Ärzteblatt International. 2021;**118**(7):109-115. Available from: https://pubmed.ncbi.nlm.nih.gov/33835006/. DOI: 10.3238/arztebl.m2021.0014

[3] Kouzy R, Abi Jaoude J, Kraitem A, El Alam MB, Karam B, Adib E, et al. Coronavirus goes viral: Quantifying the COVID-19 misinformation epidemic on twitter. Cureus. 2020;**12**(3):e7255. Available from: https://pubmed.ncbi.nlm.nih.gov/32292669/. DOI: 10.7759/cureus.7255

[4] Islam MS, Sarkar T, Khan SH, Mostofa Kamal AH, Hasan SMM, Kabir A, et al. COVID-19-related infodemic and its impact on public health: A global social media analysis. The American Journal of Tropical Medicine and Hygiene. 2020;**103**(4):1621-1629. Available from: https://pubmed.ncbi.nlm.nih.gov/32783794/. DOI: 10.4269/ajtmh.20-0812

[5] Greenstone G. The history of bloodletting. British Columbia Medical Journal. 2010;**52**(1):12-14. Available from: https://bcmj.org/premise/history-bloodletting#:~:text=By%3A%20Gerry%20Greenstone%2C%20MD%2C,a%20treatment%20for%20most%20ailments

[6] World Health Organization. Infodemic [Internet]. World Health Organization; 2025. Available from: https://www.who.int/health-topics/infodemic#tab=tab_1

[7] Ashby J. The Effects of Medical Misinformation on the American Public [Internet]. Ballard Brief; 2024. Available from: https://ballardbrief.byu.edu/issue-briefs/the-effects-of-medical-misinformation-on-the-american-public

[8] Fridman I, Johnson S, Elston LJ. Health information and misinformation: A framework to guide research and practice. JMIR Medical Education. 2023;**9**:e38687. Available from: https://www.ncbi.nlm.nih.gov/pmc/articles/PMC10285617. DOI: 10.2196/38687

[9] National Cancer Institute. Health Information National Trends Survey (HINTS). 2022. Available from: https://hints.cancer.gov/view-questions-topics/question-details.aspx?PK_Cycle=12&qid=688

[10] Johnson SB, Parsons M, Dorff T, Moran MS, Ward JH, Cohen SA, et al. Cancer misinformation and harmful information on Facebook and other social media: A brief report. Journal of the National Cancer Institute. 2021;**113**(8):1036-1039. Available from: https://pubmed.ncbi.nlm.nih.gov/34270265/. DOI: 10.1093/jnci/djab141

[11] Grande D, Shea JA, Armstrong K. Pharmaceutical industry gifts to physicians: Patient beliefs and trust in physicians and the health care system. Journal of General Internal Medicine. 2012;**27**(3):274-279. Available from: https://pubmed.ncbi.nlm.nih.gov/22006079/. DOI: 10.1007/s11606-011-1760-3

[12] Wazana A. Physicians and the pharmaceutical industry: Is a

gift ever just a gift? Journal of the American Medical Association. 2000;**283**(3):373-380. Available from: https://jamanetwork.com/journals/jama/fullarticle/192314. DOI: 10.1001/jama.283.3.373

[13] Walton A. Steve Jobs' cancer treatment regrets. Forbes. 2011. Available from: https://www.forbes.com/sites/alicegwalton/2011/10/24/steve-jobs-cancer-treatment-regrets/

[14] Kapantai E, Christopoulou A, Berberidis C, Peristeras V. A systematic literature review on disinformation: Toward a unified taxonomical framework. New Media & Society. 2021;**23**(5):1301-1326. Available from: https://journals.sagepub.com/doi/10.1177/1461444820959296. DOI: 10.1177/1461444820959296

[15] Micich A, Cross RJ. How Misinformation on Social Media has Changed News [Internet]. U.S. PIRG Education Fund; 2023. Available from: https://pirg.org/edfund/articles/misinformation-on-social-media/

[16] Molina MD, Sundar SS, Le T, Lee D. "Fake news" is not simply false information: A concept explication and taxonomy of online content. American Behavioral Scientist. 2019;**65**(2):180-212. Available from: https://journals.sagepub.com/doi/10.1177/0002764219878224. DOI: 10.1177/0002764219878224

[17] Oeberst A, Cress U. Hard facts: A meta-analysis of the anecdotal bias. Organizational Behavior and Human Decision Processes. 2020;**160**:51-67. Available from: https://www.sciencedirect.com/science/article/pii/S0749597819302933. DOI: 10.1016/j.obhdp.2020.01.001

[18] The Coronavirus Vaccines and Misinformation [Internet]. Pew.org. The Pew Charitable Trusts; 2021. Available from: https://www.pew.org/en/trust/archive/spring-2021/the-coronavirus-vaccines-and-misinformation [Accessed: October 9, 2025]

[19] Brown JD, Wissow LS, Gadomski A, Zachary C, Bartlett E, Horn I, et al. Parent and teacher mental health ratings of children: Agreement and associations with adversity. The American Journal of the Medical Sciences. 2016;**352**(6):609-616. Available from: https://www.amjmedsci.org/article/S0002-9629(15)37996-9/fulltext. DOI: 10.1016/j.amjms.2015.12.015

[20] Petryk S. In children with autism, is intravenous secretin more effective than placebo in improving social skills, communication, behaviour or global functioning? Part A: Evidence-based answer and summary. Paediatrics & Child Health. 2004;**9**(4):244-245. Available from: https://academic.oup.com/pch/article/9/4/244/2648576. DOI: 10.1093/pch/9.4.244

[21] World Health Organization. Managing the COVID-19 Infodemic: An Ad Hoc WHO Technical Consultation, Call for Action, 7-8 April 2020. Geneva: World Health Organization; 2020. Available from: https://iris.who.int/bitstream/handle/10665/334287/9789240010314-eng.pdf

[22] Guarda RF et al. Disinformation, dystopia and post-reality in social media: A semiotic-cognitive perspective. Education for Information. 2018;**34**(3):185-197. Available from: https://content.iospress.com/articles/education-for-information/efi180209. DOI: 10.3233/EFI-180209

[23] MacFarlane D et al. Refuting spurious COVID-19 treatment claims reduces demand and misinformation

sharing. Journal of Applied Research in Memory and Cognition. 2021;**10**(2):248-258. Available from: https://www.sciencedirect.com/science/article/pii/S2211368121000098. DOI: 10.1016/j.jarmac.2020.12.005

[24] Pennycook G, Rand DG. The psychology of fake news. Trends in Cognitive Sciences. 2021;**25**(5):388-402. Available from: https://www.sciencedirect.com/science/article/pii/S136466132100059X. DOI: 10.1016/j.tics.2021.02.007

[25] Miles J, Petrie C, Steel M. Slimming on the Internet. Journal of the Royal Society of Medicine. 2000;**93**(5):254-257. Available from: https://journals.sagepub.com/doi/10.1177/014107680009300509. DOI: 10.1177/014107680009300509

[26] Spurling GK, Mansfield PR, Montgomery BD, Lexchin J, Doust J, Othman N, et al. Information from pharmaceutical companies and the quality, quantity, and cost of physicians' prescribing: A systematic review. PLoS Medicine. 2010;**7**(10):e1000352. Available from: https://journals.plos.org/plosmedicine/article?id=10.1371/journal.pmed.1000352. DOI: 10.1371/journal.pmed.1000352

[27] Gagnon MA, Lexchin J. The cost of pushing pills: A new estimate of pharmaceutical promotion expenditures in the United States. PLoS Medicine. 2008;**5**(1):e1. Available from: https://journals.plos.org/plosmedicine/article?id=10.1371/journal.pmed.0050001. DOI: 10.1371/journal.pmed.0050001

[28] Fickweiler F, Fickweiler W, Urbach E. Interactions between physicians and the pharmaceutical industry generally and sales representatives specifically and their association with physicians' attitudes and prescribing habits: A systematic review. BMJ Open. 2017;**7**(9):e016408. Available from: https://bmjopen.bmj.com/content/7/9/e016408. DOI: 10.1136/bmjopen-2017-016408

[29] Piller C. Patients' mistrust of drug industry puts pressure on FDA. Science. 2020;**369**(6500):125-126. Available from: https://www.science.org/doi/10.1126/science.369.6500.125. DOI: 10.1126/science.369.6500.125

[30] Lundahl B, Kunz C, Brownell C, Tollefson D, Burke B. A meta-analysis of motivational interviewing: Twenty-five years of empirical studies. Research on Social Work Practice. 2010;**20**(2):137-160. DOI: 10.1177/1049731509347850

[31] Heckman C, Egleston B, Hofmann M. Efficacy of motivational interviewing for smoking cessation: A systematic review and meta-analysis. Tobacco Control. 2010;**19**(5):410-416. DOI: 10.1136/tc.2009.033175

[32] Barnes R, Ivezaj V. A systematic review of motivational interviewing for weight loss among adults in primary care. Obesity Reviews. 2015;**16**(4):304-318. DOI: 10.1111/obr.12264

[33] Cascaes A, Bielemann R, Clark V, Barros A. Effectiveness of motivational interviewing at improving oral health: A systematic review. Revista de Saúde Pública. 2014;**48**(1):142-153. DOI: 10.1590/s0034-8910.2014048004616

[34] Mose L, Bornhøft J, Primdahl J, Gram B. Coping and motivation for change—An interview study of the experience from participation in an educational program for patients with medication-overuse headache. Journal of Patient Experience. 1 Jan 2021;**8**:237437352110342. DOI: 10.1177/23743735211034289

[35] Westra H, Aviram A. Core skills in motivational interviewing. Psychotherapy. 2013;**50**(3):273-278. DOI: 10.1037/a0032409

[36] Schechter N, Butt L, Jacocks C, Staguhn ED, Castillo RC, Wegener ST. Evaluation of an online motivational interviewing training program for rehabilitation professionals: A pilot study. Clinical Rehabilitation. 2021;**35**(9):1266-1276. DOI: 10.1177/02692155211002958

[37] Suárez-Lledó V, Álvarez-Gálvez J. Prevalence of health misinformation on social media: Systematic review. Journal of Medical Internet Research. 2021;**23**(1):e17187. DOI: 10.2196/17187

[38] Chou W, Oh A, Klein W. Addressing health-related misinformation on social media. JAMA. 2018;**320**(23):2417. DOI: 10.1001/jama.2018.16865

[39] Lip A, Pateman M, Fullerton MM, Chen HM, Bailey L, Houle S, et al. Vaccine hesitancy educational tools for healthcare providers and trainees: A scoping review. Vaccine. 2023;**41**(1):23-35. DOI: 10.1016/j.vaccine.2022.09.093

[40] Schneider-Kamp A, Takhar J. Interrogating the pill: Rising distrust and the reshaping of health risk perceptions in the social media age. Social Science & Medicine. 2023;**331**:116081. DOI: 10.1016/j.socscimed.2023.116081

[41] Brewer NT. What works to increase vaccination uptake. Academic Pediatrics. 2021;**21**(4 Suppl):S9-S16. DOI: 10.1016/j.acap.2021.01.017

[42] Limaye RJ, Opel DJ, Dempsey A, Ellingson M, Spina C, Omer SB, et al. Communicating with vaccine-hesitant parents: A narrative review. Academic Pediatrics. 2021;**21**(4 Suppl):S24-S29. DOI: 10.1016/j.acap.2021.01.018. Erratum in: Academic Pediatrics 2023; 23(4), 849. doi: 10.1016/j.acap.2021.08.002

[43] Kammering H, Cruz JA, Platzbecker AL, Reinauer C, Förtsch K, Krassuski L, et al. Motivational interview from the paediatricians' perspective: Assessments after a 2-day training for physicians caring for adolescents with chronic medical conditions (CMCs). BMC Pediatrics. 2024;**24**(1):355. DOI: 10.1186/s12887-024-04794-z

[44] Løchting I, Hagen R, Monsen CK, Grotle M, Storheim K, Aanesen F, et al. Fidelity of a motivational interviewing intervention for improving return to work for people with musculoskeletal disorders. International Journal of Environmental Research and Public Health. 2021;**18**(19):10324. DOI: 10.3390/ijerph181910324

[45] Chakrapani V, Kaur M, Tsai AC, Newman PA, Kumar R. The impact of a syndemic theory-based intervention on HIV transmission risk behaviour among men who have sex with men in India: Pretest-posttest non-equivalent comparison group trial. Social Science & Medicine. 2022;**295**:112817. DOI: 10.1016/j.socscimed.2020.112817

[46] Meng DF, Bao J, Cai TZ, Ji YJ, Yang Y. Music therapy combined with motivational interviewing. World Journal of Psychiatry. 2024;**14**(12):1886-1891. DOI: 10.5498/wjp.v14.i12.1886

[47] MacDonald NE. Fake news and science denier attacks on vaccines. What can you do? Canada Communicable Disease Report. 2020;**46**(11-12):432-435. DOI: 10.14745/ccdr.v46i1112a11

[48] Franklin BA, Myers J, Kokkinos P. Importance of lifestyle modification on cardiovascular risk reduction: Counselling strategies to maximize patient outcomes. Journal of

Cardiopulmonary Rehabilitation and Prevention. 2020;**40**(3):138-143. DOI: 10.1097/HCR.0000000000000496

[49] Holford D, Schmid P, Fasce A, Lewandowsky S. The empathetic refutational interview to tackle vaccine misconceptions: Four randomized experiments. Health Psychology. 2024;**43**(6):426-437. DOI: 10.1037/hea0001354

[50] Ismail N, Kbaier Ben Ismail D, Farrell T, Kane A. The experience of health professionals with misinformation and its impact on their job practice: Qualitative interview study. JMIR Formative Research. 2022;**6**:e38794. DOI: 10.2196/38794

[51] Gong SA, Ao SH, Chen YS. The influence of patient-centered communication on psychological distress: The chain mediating role of health-related self-efficacy and healthy lifestyle behaviors and the moderating role of social media use. Frontiers in Psychiatry. 2025;**16**:1562414. DOI: 10.3389/fpsyt.2025.1562414

[52] McIntyre H, Reeves V, Loughhead M, Hayes L, Procter N. Communication pathways from the emergency department to community mental health services: A systematic review. International Journal of Mental Health Nursing. 2022;**31**(6):1282-1299. DOI: 10.1111/inm.13024

[53] Arnett MC, Paulson DR, Evans MD, Blue CM, Reibel YG. Health topics emerged from brief-motivational interviewing: A randomized clinical trial. International Journal of Dental Hygiene. 2023;**21**(4):738-746. DOI: 10.1111/idh.12739

[54] Olson O, Berry C, Kumar N. Addressing parental vaccine hesitancy towards childhood vaccines in the United States: A systematic literature review of communication interventions and strategies. Vaccines (Basel). 2020;**8**(4):590. DOI: 10.3390/vaccines8040590

[55] Akinrolie O, Strachan S, Webber SC, Chan H, Messner K, Barclay R. Counsellors' verbal behaviours and skills that elicit participants' change or sustain talk in virtual motivational interviewing for physical activity among older adults. Applied Psychology. Health and Well-Being. 2024;**16**(4):1699-1715. DOI: 10.1111/aphw.12551

[56] Lentz C, Giguere R, Kutner BA, Dolezal C, Kajura-Manyindo C, Yambira M, et al. Culturally-based challenges to and recommendations for delivering adherence counseling in a multicultural biomedical HIV prevention trial in four African countries. AIDS Education and Prevention. 2020;**32**(6):512-527. DOI: 10.1521/aeap.2020.32.6.512

[57] Opel DJ, Robinson JD, Zhou C, et al. Tiered clinician vaccine communication strategy to improve childhood vaccine uptake: A cluster randomized clinical trial. JAMA Network Open. 2025;**8**(4):e257814. DOI: 10.1001/jamanetworkopen.2025.7814

[58] Tanaka A, Aggarwal S, Arena R, Wang M, Liang Z, Campbell T, et al. The potential influence of depressive symptoms on outcomes from a brief motivational intervention in patients referred to cardiac rehabilitation. Patient Education and Counseling. 2025;**138**:109206. DOI: 10.1016/j.pec.2025.109206

[59] Muyambi K, Walsh S, Bressington D, Gray R, Dennis S, Brown E, et al. Efficacy of behavioural activation in the treatment of negative symptoms in people with schizophrenia spectrum

disorders: A systematic review. International Journal of Nursing Studies Advances. 2023;**5**:100132. DOI: 10.1016/j.ijnsa.2023.100132

[60] Ramirez MR, Flores JE, Woods-Jaeger B, Cavanaugh JE, Peek-Asa C, Branch C, et al. Comparative effectiveness of parent-based interventions to support injured children. Pediatrics. 2021;**148**(4):e2020046920. DOI: 10.1542/peds.2020-046920

[61] Thongsunti A, Silpakit C, Rattananupong T, Kittanamongkolchai W, Sumethpimolchai W, Lohsoonthorn V. Effect of a transtheoretical model-based intervention and motivational interviewing on hyperphosphatemia management via telehealth (TMT program) among hemodialysis patients during the COVID-19 pandemic. Frontiers in Public Health. 2024;**12**:1361778. DOI: 10.3389/fpubh.2024.1361778

[62] Pérula-Jiménez C, Romero-Rodríguez E, Parras-Rejano JM, de la Rubia AG, Gómez JB, de Torres LAP, et al. Effectiveness of a training program for the management of risky alcohol use in primary care professionals based on motivational interviewing. Atencion Primaria. 2024;**56**(4):102835. DOI: 10.1016/j.aprim.2023.102835

[63] Khedr MA, Ali EA, Sanhoury MI, Hussein RM. The feasibility of motivational interviewing on adherence to care practices, emotional intelligence, and dispositional optimism among patients with permanent pacemakers. European Journal of Cardiovascular Nursing. 2024;**23**(5):497-509. DOI: 10.1093/eurjcn/zvad113

[64] Wang L, Li J, Zhang M, Chan MMK, Ho MH. Effectiveness of transtheoretical model-based motivational interviewing on glycemic control among adults with type 2 diabetes: A systematic review and meta-analysis of randomized control trials. Worldviews on Evidence-Based Nursing. 2025;**22**(3):e70041. DOI: 10.1111/wvn.70041

[65] Dubov A, Distelberg BJ, Abdul-Mutakabbir JC, Beeson WL, Loo LK, Montgomery SB, et al. Predictors of COVID-19 vaccine acceptance and hesitancy among healthcare workers in Southern California: Not just "anti" vs. "pro" vaccine. Vaccines (Basel). 2021;**9**(12):1428. DOI: 10.3390/vaccines9121428

[66] Fasce A, Mustață M, Deliu A, et al. A field test of empathetic refutational and motivational interviewing to address vaccine hesitancy among patients. npj Vaccines. 2025;**10**:142. DOI: 10.1038/s41541-025-01197-8

[67] Dumitra GG, Camen AR, Nechita F, Pîrlog MC, Kamal C, Dogaru CA, et al. Effectiveness of group and individual counselling interventions on COVID-19 vaccination intention among industrial employees in Romania. Patient Preference and Adherence. 2025;**19**:907-919. DOI: 10.2147/PPA.S500640

[68] Perkins JR, Jaqua EE, Nguyen VT, Franz DA, Elkins J, Morton KR. Optimizing education to improve COVID-19 vaccination rates in a federally qualified health center. The Permanente Journal. 2023;**27**(4):143-150. DOI: 10.7812/TPP/23.088

[69] Lim C, Van Alphen MU, Maclaurin S, Mulligan C, Macri B, Cather C, et al. Increasing COVID-19 vaccination rates among patients with serious mental illness: A pilot intervention study. Psychiatric Services. 2022;**73**(11):1274-1277. DOI: 10.1176/appi.ps.202100702

[70] Aubeeluck E, Al-Arkee S, Finlay K, Jalal Z. The impact of pharmacy care and motivational interviewing on improving

medication adherence in patients with cardiovascular diseases: A systematic review of randomized controlled trials. International Journal of Clinical Practice. 2021;**75**(11):e14457. DOI: 10.1111/ijcp.14457

[71] Wandscher K, Hoffmann F, Heesen C, Thomalla G, Rahn AC, Helbach J. Effectiveness of motivational interviewing on medication adherence for the prevention of recurrent stroke or transient ischemic attack: Systematic review of randomized controlled trials. European Journal of Neurology. 2024;**31**(8):e16313. DOI: 10.1111/ene.16313

[72] Melnick R, Mendonça CS, Meyer E, Faustino-Silva DD. Effectiveness of motivational interviewing in smoking groups in primary healthcare: A community-based randomized cluster trial. Cadernos De Saude Publica. 2021;**37**(3):e00038820. DOI: 10.1590/0102-311X00038820

[73] Olusanya OA, Masters NB, Zhang F, Sugerman DE, Carter RJ, Weiss D, et al. Sociodemographic trends and correlation between parental hesitancy towards pediatric COVID-19 vaccines and routine childhood immunizations in the United States: 2021-2022 national immunization survey-child COVID module. Vaccines (Basel). 3 May 2024;**12**(5):495. DOI: 10.3390/vaccines12050495

[74] Kaushik A, Fomicheva J, Boonstra N, Faber E, Gupta S, Kest H. Pediatric vaccine hesitancy in the United States—The growing problem and strategies for management including motivational interviewing. Vaccines (Basel). 2025;**13**(2):115. Available from: https://www.mdpi.com/2076-393X/13/2/115. DOI: 10.3390/vaccines13020115

[75] Austin EW, O'Donnell N, Rose P, Edwards Z, Sheftel A, Domgaard S, et al. Integrating science media literacy, motivational interviewing, and neuromarketing science to increase vaccine education confidence among U.S. extension professionals. Vaccines (Basel). 2024;**12**(8):869. Available from: https://www.mdpi.com/2076-393X/12/8/869. DOI: 10.3390/vaccines12080869

[76] Brehm JW. Psychological reactance: Theory and applications. Advances in Consumer Research [Internet]. 1 Jan 1989;**16**(1):72-75. Available from: https://research.ebsco.com/linkprocessor/plink?id=47c5a90e-ff6e-343e-a60a-3d0f6764014e [Accessed: October 9, 2025]

[77] Scales D, Gorman JM, DiCaprio P, Hurth L, Radhakrishnan M, Windham S, et al. Community-oriented motivational interviewing (MI): A novel framework extending MI to address COVID-19 vaccine misinformation in online social media platforms. Computers in Human Behavior. Apr 2023;**141**:107609. DOI: 10.1016/j.chb.2022.107609. Epub 2022 Dec 13

[78] Lapane KL, Dubé CE, Schneider KL, Quilliam BJ. Misperceptions of patients vs providers regarding medication-related communication issues. The American Journal of Managed Care. 2007;**13**(10):613-618. Available from: https://pubmed.ncbi.nlm.nih.gov/17988182/

[79] Krueger KP, Berger BA, Felkey B. Medication adherence and persistence: A comprehensive review. Advances in Therapy. 2005;**22**(4):313-356. Available from: https://pubmed.ncbi.nlm.nih.gov/16418141/. DOI: 10.1007/BF02850081

[80] Marcum ZA, Gellad WF. Medication adherence to multidrug regimens. Clinics in Geriatric Medicine. 2012;**28**(2):287-300. Available

from: https://pubmed.ncbi.nlm.nih.gov/22500544/. DOI: 10.1016/j.cger.2012.01.008

[81] Kempe A, Saville AW, Albertin C, Zimet G, Breck A, Helmkamp L, et al. Parental hesitancy about routine childhood and influenza vaccinations: A national survey. Pediatrics. 2020;**146**(1):e20193852. Available from: https://publications.aap.org/pediatrics/article/146/1/e20193852/37164/Parental-Hesitancy-About-Routine-Childhood-and. DOI: 10.1542/peds.2019-3852

[82] Dana J, Loewenstein G. A social science perspective on gifts to physicians from industry. Journal of the American Medical Association. 2003;**290**(2):252-255. Available from: https://jamanetwork.com/journals/jama/fullarticle/196342. DOI: 10.1001/jama.290.2.252

[83] Carroll AE, Vreeman RC. Pharmaceutical gifts to physicians: Patient and physician perceptions. BMJ. 2005;**330**(7486):409-410. Available from: https://www.bmj.com/content/330/7486/409. DOI: 10.1136/bmj.330.7486.409

[84] Ziegler MG, Lew P, Singer BC. The accuracy of drug information from pharmaceutical sales representatives. Journal of the American Medical Association. 1995;**273**(16):1296-1298. Available from: https://jamanetwork.com/journals/jama/fullarticle/387015. DOI: 10.1001/jama.1995.03520360054034

[85] Zhu SF, Sinha D, Kirk M, Michalopoulou M, Hajizadeh A, Wren G, et al. Effectiveness of behavioural interventions with motivational interviewing on physical activity outcomes in adults: Systematic review and meta-analysis. BMJ. 2024;**386**:e078713. DOI: 10.1136/bmj-2023-078713

[86] Norris P, Herxheimer A, Lexchin J, Mansfield P. Drug Promotion: What we Know, What we Have Yet to Learn. Geneva: World Health Organization; 2005. Available from: https://apps.who.int/iris/handle/10665/69177

[87] Segado Fernández S, Jiménez Gómez B, Jiménez Hidalgo P, Lozano-Estevan MDC, Herrera PI. Disinformation about diet and nutrition on social networks: A review of the literature. Nutricion Hospitalaria. 2025;**42**(2):366-375. Available from: https://scielo.isciii.es/scielo.php?script=sci_arttext&pid=S0212-16112025000200366. DOI: 10.20960/nh.05533

[88] Diekman C, Ryan CD, Oliver TL. Misinformation and disinformation in food science and nutrition: Impact on practice. The Journal of Nutrition. 2023;**153**(1):3-9. Available from: https://www.sciencedirect.com/science/article/pii/S0022316622010216. DOI: 10.1016/j.tjnut.2022.10.001

[89] World Health Organization. Ten Threats to Global Health in 2019. Geneva: WHO; 2019. Available from: https://www.who.int/news-room/spotlight/ten-threats-to-global-health-in-2019

[90] Fugh-Berman A, Ahari S. Following the script: How drug reps make friends and influence doctors. PLoS Medicine. 2007;**4**(4):e150. Available from: https://journals.plos.org/plosmedicine/article?id=10.1371/journal.pmed.0040150. DOI: 10.1371/journal.pmed.0040150

[91] Swartz HA, Zuckoff A, Frank E, Spielvogle HN, Grote NK, Bledsoe SE, et al. An

open-label trial of enhanced brief interpersonal psychotherapy in depressed mothers whose children are receiving psychiatric treatment. Depression and Anxiety. 2006;**23**(7):398-404. Available from: https://onlinelibrary.wiley.com/doi/10.1002/da.20179. DOI: 10.1002/da.20179

[92] Van Voorhees BW, Fogel J, Reinecke MA, Gladstone T, Stuart S, Gollan J, et al. Randomized clinical trial of an Internet-based depression prevention program for adolescents (Project CATCH-IT) in primary care: 12-week outcomes. Journal of Developmental and Behavioral Pediatrics. 2009;**30**(1):23-37. Available from: https://journals.lww.com/jrnldbp/Fulltext/2009/02000/Randomized_Clinical_Trial_of_an_Internet_Based.4.aspx. DOI: 10.1097/DBP.0b013e3181966c2a

[93] Pung MA. Motivational interview in the reduction of risk factors for eating disorders: A pilot study. Dissertation Abstracts International: Section B: The Sciences and Engineering. 2004;**65**:3178. Available from: https://www.proquest.com/openview/11aadb0dce9a9a6af1f8a7af7b96f1d7/1

[94] Grundy Q, Bero L, Malone R. Interactions between non-physician clinicians and industry: A systematic review. PLoS Medicine. 2013;**10**(11):e1001561. Available from: https://journals.plos.org/plosmedicine/article?id=10.1371/journal.pmed.1001561. DOI: 10.1371/journal.pmed.1001561

[95] Steinberg ML, Ziedonis DM, Krejci JA, Brandon TH. Motivational interview with personalized feedback: A brief intervention for motivating smokers with schizophrenia to seek treatment for tobacco dependence. Journal of Consulting and Clinical Psychology. 2004;**72**(4):723-728. Available from: https://psycnet.apa.org/doi/10.1037/0022-006X.72.4.723. DOI: 10.1037/0022-006X.72.4.723

[96] Kemp R, Hayward P, Applewhaite G, Everitt B, David A. Compliance therapy in psychotic patients: Randomised controlled trial. BMJ. 1996;**312**(7027):345-349. Available from: https://www.bmj.com/content/312/7027/345. DOI: 10.1136/bmj.312.7027.345

[97] Kemp R, Kirov G, Everitt B, Hayward P, David AS. Randomised controlled trial of compliance therapy. 18-month follow-up. The British Journal of Psychiatry. 1998;**172**(5):413-419. Available from: https://www.cambridge.org/core/journals/the-british-journal-of-psychiatry/article/randomised-controlled-trial-of-compliance-therapy-18month-followup/16BB8AD711A5DF4CCB393C857E508BE3. DOI: 10.1192/bjp.172.5.413

[98] McCambridge J, Strang J. The efficacy of single-session motivational interviewing in reducing drug consumption and perceptions of drug-related risk and harm among young people: Results from a multi-site cluster randomized trial. Addiction. 2004;**99**(1):39-52. Available from: https://onlinelibrary.wiley.com/doi/10.1111/j.1360-0443.2004.00564.x. DOI: 10.1111/j.1360-0443.2004.00564.x

[99] Forman DP, Moyers TB. With odds of a single session, motivational interviewing is a good bet. Psychotherapy (Chicago, Ill.). 2019;**56**(1):62-66. Available from: https://psycnet.apa.org/doi/10.1037/pst0000199. DOI: 10.1037/pst0000199

[100] Silverman J, Kurtz S, Draper J. Skills for Communicating with Patients. 3rd ed. Boca Raton (FL): CRC Press; 2013.

Available from: https://www.routledge.com/Skills-for-Communicating-with-Patients/Silverman-Kurtz-Draper/p/book/9781138030253. DOI: 10.1201/b13446

[101] Ford C, Hasan H, Fullerton M, Wong J, Pateman M, Chen HM, et al. Leveraging Canadian health care worker volunteers to address COVID-19 vaccine misinformation on Facebook: Qualitative program evaluation study. Journal of medical Internet research [Internet]. 2025;**27**:e65361. Available from: https://pubmed.ncbi.nlm.nih.gov/40705481/ DOI: 10.2196/65361.

Chapter 9

Perspective Chapter: Management of a Patient Complaining of Vertigo or Dizziness in General Practice

Michalina Piechocka and Przemysław Śpiewak

Abstract

This chapter provides a comprehensive overview of the symptomatology associated with the most common vestibular disorders encountered in general practice, including Benign Paroxysmal Positional Vertigo, Vestibular Migraine, Vestibular Neuritis, and Ménière's disease. It discusses the population prevalence of vertigo and dizziness, highlighting their significance as prevalent symptoms in various age groups. The text also addresses vertigo and dizziness as potential adverse drug reactions, emphasizing the importance of medication history in diagnosis. Differentiation between peripheral and central causes of vertigo is explored through detailed clinical interviews and physical examination findings, aiding in accurate diagnosis. Additionally, strategies for providing immediate symptomatic relief to patients experiencing dizziness or vertigo are outlined. The chapter delineates criteria for urgent hospital referral, identifying red flags that necessitate prompt investigation. Furthermore, it clarifies the appropriate specialist referrals, distinguishing cases requiring otolaryngological assessment from those needing neurological evaluation, to optimize patient management and outcomes.

Keywords: vertigo, dizziness, vestibular assessment, otolaryngologist, neurologist

1. Introduction

Vertigo, dizziness, and gait instability are among the most prevalent and diagnostically challenging symptoms encountered in primary care settings. These sensations can markedly impair a patient's quality of life, with etiologies ranging from benign vestibular disturbances to potentially life-threatening neurological or systemic conditions. As the initial point of medical contact, the general practitioner plays a pivotal role in the preliminary assessment, diagnostic evaluation, and management of patients presenting with these symptoms. Recognizing red flags and understanding indications for urgent intervention or specialist referral are critical for delivering effective patient care.

2. Epidemiology of dizziness and balance disorders

Dizziness and balance disorders, collectively referred to as Vertigo, Dizziness, and Unsteadiness (VDU), are prevalent symptoms associated with vestibular dysfunction and are among the most common reasons for patients to seek medical attention [1–3]. According to national surveys conducted over a 1-year period, the annual prevalence of these symptoms within the population ranges from 14.8 to 35.6% [3–8]. The likelihood of experiencing VDU increases with advancing age, reaching approximately 45% in individuals over 65 years and rising to as high as 54% among those aged 80 and older [2, 5, 8, 9].

VDU significantly heightens the risk of falls that can result in injuries and adversely affects the quality of life for those affected. This situation imposes considerable financial burdens on both patients and national healthcare systems [2–5, 9–15]. Neuhauser reports that nearly 80% of patients presenting with vertigo of the "Vertigo" type seek medical consultation and often require temporary sick leave [5]. In urban populations in London and Siena, chronic or recurrent dizziness has led to 21% of respondents discontinuing their previous employment, while 27% modified the nature of their professional responsibilities. Additionally, approximately 50% of individuals experiencing VDU reported a decline in work productivity. Furthermore, around 57% of respondents noted a deterioration in their social quality of life, and 30% indicated challenges in familial relationships. More than 50% of study participants expressed a reluctance to travel due to their symptoms [13].

Estimating the precise prevalence of disorders and defects of the peripheral vestibular system is inherently challenging. Despite this issue's widespread nature, experts estimate that approximately 80% of people worldwide experiencing "vertigo" or "dizziness" remain undiagnosed. The lack of standardized protocols for the management of patients with VDU contributes to unnecessary diagnostic testing and, more critically, impedes the implementation of effective treatment strategies [15].

The organization of care for patients with VDU is further complicated by the fact that symptoms such as dizziness and instability may arise from not only lesions within the labyrinth or cerebellum but also from dysfunctions within the motor and proprioceptive systems, visual pathways, and other neurological pathways. The functionality of these systems is influenced by the efficacy of the cardiovascular, respiratory, and metabolic systems, including hepatic, renal, and pancreatic functions. Additionally, central modulation and inhibition of vestibular activity may be disrupted during episodes of acute stress, panic attacks, and other mental health disorders. Considering the diverse and multifactorial etiology of VDU, patients presenting with these symptoms may require management by healthcare professionals from various specialties, as well as non-medical practitioners, as detailed in **Table 1**.

It is presumed that the most prevalent causes of vertigo and dizziness are related to impairments of the peripheral vestibular system [1–5, 8]. Unfortunately, there is currently no quantitative method available to assess the excitability threshold of the vestibular organ in patients, analogous to the use of tonal audiometry for the auditory system. Furthermore, it is not feasible to stimulate the vestibular system using stimuli of varying intensity and frequency while objectively recording the subject's responses [16].

Healthcare professionals engaged in the care of patients with VDU	
Physicians	**Non-physicians**
• General Practitioner • Otolaryngologist • Audiovestibular Physician • Neurologist • Rehabilitation Specialist • Emergency Medicine Specialist • Ophthalmologist • Psychiatrist • Geriatrician • Cardiologist • Angiologist • Vascular Surgeon	• Physiotherapist • Audiologist • Psychologist • Nurse • Paramedic • Physician assistant • Optometrist • Medical physicist

Table 1.
Healthcare professionals engaged in the care of patients with VDU.

3. Symptoms

Symptoms such as vertigo and dizziness are among the most prevalent reasons for patients to seek consultation from primary care physicians. Survey studies indicate that between 14.8% and 35.6% of respondents have reported experiencing these symptoms within a one-year period [1–4]. The prevalence of dizziness is observed to increase with advancing age and is more frequently reported by women compared to men. This condition may affect over 50% of individuals aged 79 years and older [1, 5, 6].

The following tables provide a comprehensive overview of vertigo, dizziness, and related sensations, along with their most common etiologies (**Table 2**), medications that may precipitate symptoms described by patients as dizziness (**Table 3**), and the duration of vertigo episodes associated with various conditions (**Table 4**). This information may prove valuable in the diagnostic assessment of VDU.

Type of discomfort	Possible cause
Vertigo refers to the sensation of spinning either of the patient's body or the surrounding environment.	• Dysfunction of the peripheral vestibular system • Vestibular paroxysms • Vestibular migraine
Dizziness is characterized by a sensation of motion, which may include feelings of the ground undulating, the perception of the surrounding environment shifting or sinking, and a sensation of the body floating.	• Central vestibular syndrome • General circulatory failure as well as in the central nervous system • Metabolic disorders due to liver, kidney, and pancreatic failure (diabetes) and other • Adverse drug reactions • Dysfunction of the visual system

Type of discomfort	Possible cause
Presyncope – fainting.	• Cardiovascular (e.g., cardiac arrhythmias) • Central (e.g., orthostatic hypotension, neuroglycopenia) • Vasovagal – parasympathetic activation
Light-headedness refers to a sensation of emptiness within the head or a sense of spatial disorientation, occurring without any accompanying perception of movement.	• Mental disorders (panic attacks, post-traumatic stress disorder (PTSD), obsessive-compulsive disorders, phobias) • Metabolic disorders
Unsteadiness – unbalance.	• Damage to the vestibular system. • Damage to the locomotor system. • Impairment of proprioception. • Defects and diseases of the visual system. • Defects and diseases of the central nervous system.

Table 2.
Vertigo, dizziness, and similar sensations and their most common causes.

Class of drugs	Active substances that may induce dizziness as an adverse effect
Statins	Atorvastatin, simvastatin
Non-opioid analgesics	Ibuprofen, celecoxib, diclofenac, naproxen, acetylsalicylic acid, paracetamol
Antidepressants	Mirtazapine, paroxetine, sertraline, amitriptyline, doxepin, trazodone
Fluoroquinolones	Ciprofloxacin, levofloxacin
Macrolides	Clarithromycin, azithromycin
ACE inhibitors	Zofenopril, enalapril
ARBs	Irbesartan
Calcium channel blockers	Amlodipine, lacidipine
Azole antifungals	Itraconazole, fluconazole
Antipsychotics	Clozapine
Dopaminergic drugs	Bromocriptine, levodopa

Table 3.
Medications that most commonly may induce symptoms described by patients as dizziness, based on Woron et al. [17].

4. Physical examination

The primary care physician should assess whether the symptoms reported by the patient are associated with balance impairment and perform posture and gait evaluations. The most widely recognized postural assessment is the Romberg test. In this test, it is recommended that the patient stand barefoot with their feet together, arms positioned either at their sides or crossed over their chest. The Romberg test is deemed normal if the individual can maintain balance for 1 minute with their eyes closed (**Figure 1**).

Duration of VDU episodes	Most common causes
Seconds	• *Benign paroxysmal positional vertigo* (BPPV) associated with the displacement of otoliths from the utricle into the semicircular canals. • *Orthostatic hypotension.* • *Vestibular paroxysmia*, often resulting from a conflict between the vestibulocochlear nerve and blood vessels in the posterior cranial fossa. • *Otolith crisis of Tumarkin (Drop Attack)*, a rare variant of Ménière's disease characterized by sudden falls without loss of consciousness. • *Perilymphatic fistula*, in the context of the third window syndrome. • *Vestibular aura*, observed as a symptom of temporal lobe epilepsy.
Minutes	• *Vestibular migraine* (duration of 5 minutes). • *Meniere's disease* (duration of 20 minutes). • *Vertebrobasilar transient ischemic attacks.* • *Episodic ataxia type 2* with cerebellar symptoms. • *Panic attack.*
Hours and days	• *Ménière's disease* (duration up to 24 hours). • *Vestibular migraine* (duration up to 72 hours). • *Mal de Débarquement syndrome (MdDS)*, a disorder characterized by non-vertiginous dizziness with a sensation of swaying or rocking, which occurs within 48 hours after the end of a journey and lasts for more than 2 days.
Weeks	• *Vestibular neuritis* is defined as an acute dysfunction of the vestibular system, characterized by a sudden onset of vertigo and associated autonomic symptoms, while lacking any auditory symptoms. The clinical manifestations typically resolve gradually over a span of several weeks to a few months. • *Persistent MdDS*
Months	• *Persistent Postural-Perceptual Dizziness (PPPD)* is a chronic disorder often preceded by other vestibular disorders. It is characterized by sensations of spatial discomfort and imbalance, particularly during standing and ambulation. This condition may persist for three months or longer

Table 4.
The duration of VDU episodes across different clinical conditions [18–26].

The Romberg test is a clinical assessment utilized to diagnose ataxia, a condition characterized by impaired coordination and balance. Ataxia may arise from various etiologies, including damage to the dorsal columns of the spinal cord (specifically the posterior column-medial lemniscus pathway), the cerebellum, and the vestibular system. The dorsal columns are responsible for transmitting critical sensory information related to proprioception from deep sensory organs to the brain, which is essential for maintaining equilibrium.

A positive Romberg sign indicates the patient's inability to maintain balance during the test and may be associated with the following conditions:

- Loss of proprioception due to myelopathy or sensory neuropathies.
- Uncompensated damage to the vestibular system.
- Cerebellar pathologies.

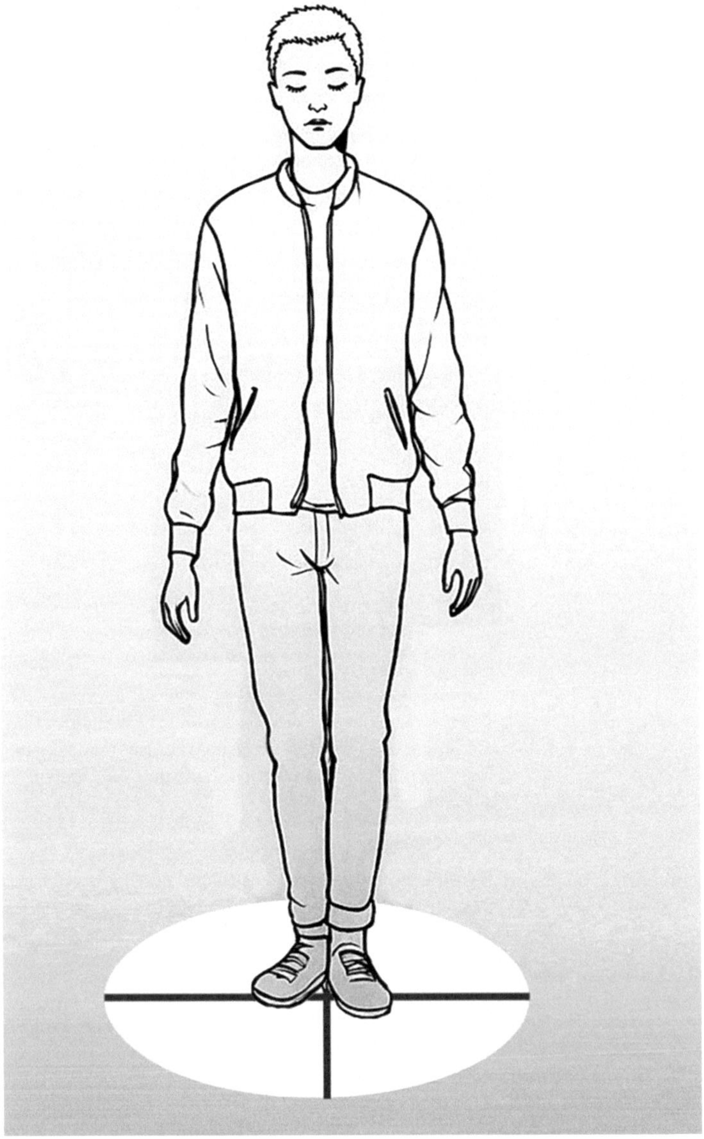

Figure 1.
The Romberg test.

In cases of uncompensated vestibular deficits, the patient tends to fall toward the affected labyrinth. Conversely, individuals with cerebellar damage often struggle to maintain balance even when their eyes are open [27]. **Table 5** provides a summary of the clinical conditions associated with an abnormal Romberg test.

The Fukuda Unterberger Stepping Test (FST) serves as a more specific assessment for vestibular dysfunction. In Europe, this test is commonly referred to as the Unterberger test, while in the United States and Asia, it is known as the Fukuda test. The FST evaluates the subjective perception of the individual's body alignment when facing straight ahead (subjective straight ahead), which is contingent upon the proper functioning of the otolithic organs located in the utricle and saccule, as well as the integrity of the central vestibular system. During the FST, the patient performs alternating steps in place with their eyes closed and arms extended forward. The test is deemed pathological if the angle of arm deviation from the initial position exceeds 30° after 50 steps or 45° after 100 steps. In instances of vestibular weakness, the patient is likely to veer toward the side of the affected labyrinth (**Figure 2**) [28–30].

Lateralization toward the affected vestibule (ipsilateralization) primarily occurs in acute cases. In chronic vestibular dysfunction, however, patients may also exhibit

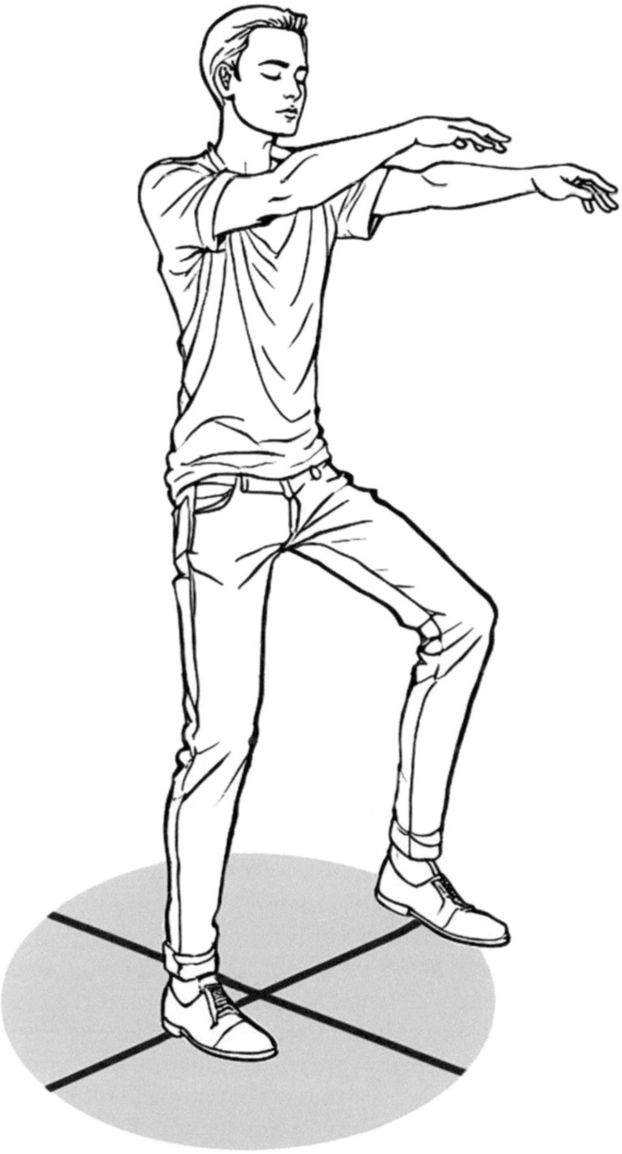

Figure 2.
The Fukuda Unterberger stepping test.

Condition	Main differentiating features
• Acute vestibular deficit • Unilateral vestibulopathy/ vestibular neuronitis • Attack of Ménière's disease (MD) • Labyrinthitis	• Nystagmus • Autonomic symptoms • In MD and labyrinthitis: hearing loss, a feeling of fullness in the ear, and tinnitus in the affected ear.
• Parkinson's disease	• Unsteadiness, "shuffling" gait
• Friedreich's ataxia	• Unsteady gait, tendency to fall
• Wernicke's syndrome	• A consequence of chronic alcoholism characterized by ataxia
• Vitamin B12 deficiency	• Atactic movements
• Tertiary syphilis	• Sensory ataxia, loss of proprioception
• Normal-pressure hydrocephalus in elderly individuals	• Truncal ataxia and episodes of falls

Table 5.
Clinical conditions associated with abnormal results in the romberg test.

a tendency to deviate toward the healthy labyrinth [31]. This alteration in the direction of deviation during the FST can be attributed to the phenomenon of vestibular compensation [32]. When evaluating a patient with acute vestibular damage at the bedside, it is important to recognize that the patient may exhibit a tendency to deviate in a direction that aligns with their previous body position, which can be significantly influenced by their prior whole-body roll orientation. For instance, a patient who has been lying on their left side for at least 5 minutes prior to the examination is likely to deviate to the left during the FST [33]. Additionally, in clinical practice, we frequently observe marked deviations in the FST among individuals with locomotor system dysfunctions—particularly those affecting the spine, hip joints, and lower limbs—even in the absence of vestibular dysfunction.

5. Characteristics of vestibular nystagmus

As stated in the introduction, the vestibular organ serves as the receptor in the vestibulo-ocular reflex (VOR), with the eye acting as the effector. The primary function of the VOR is to stabilize the image on the retina. When functional asymmetry occurs between the vestibular systems, involuntary and rhythmic eye movements, referred to as nystagmus, emerge. Vestibular nystagmus exhibits a coordinated nature, characterized by simultaneous movement of both eyes in the same direction and with identical amplitude. This phenomenon consists of two phases: a fast phase and a slow phase. The direction of the fast phase indicates the more stimulated, or typically better functioning, vestibular system. Observationally, the eye movements are predominantly horizontal or rotational. Fixation of gaze serves to inhibit vestibular nystagmus. Following a sudden loss of vestibular function, the intensity of nystagmus gradually diminishes and ultimately resolves upon completion of the vestibular compensation process [34, 35]. Refer to **Table 6** for further details.

Vestibular nystagmus	Non-vestibular nystagmus (central or ocular)
Always gathered	In central nervous system (CNS) injuries, it may be ungathered
Biphasic with fast and slow phases	It may be oscillatory (especially ocular)
In a consistent direction, irrespective of the line of sight	In CNS disorders, a change in the direction of gaze can alter the direction of nystagmus
Most often horizontal or horizontal-rotary in an 'unarmed eye' examination	Eyeballs are capable of movement within the vertical and oblique planes, or others
Fixation of gaze reduces the intensity of the symptom	No effect of fixation of gaze on the intensity of nystagmus
After the sudden loss of vestibular function, the severity of symptoms gradually decreases over time	It may intensify or weaken over time

Table 6.
Differentiating vestibular nystagmus from non-vestibular nystagmus.

6. The HINTS examination: Differentiation of acute vestibular syndrome (AVS) from posterior cranial fossa stroke

In the preliminary examination, the symptoms observed during the initial hours of acute vestibular syndrome (AVS), specifically vestibular neuronitis (VN), and strokes originating from arteries branching off the vertebral or basilar arteries in the posterior cranial fossa exhibit considerable similarities. Both conditions present with severe vertiginous symptoms, accompanied by pronounced nystagmus and autonomic symptoms such as vomiting and nausea. However, the clinical outcomes of these conditions differ significantly. In cases of AVS, symptoms typically resolve spontaneously over time, warranting only symptomatic management, which may include the administration of antiemetics and the replenishment of lost fluids and electrolytes. Conversely, in the event of a stroke, it is imperative that the patient be transferred to a medical facility for treatment as soon as possible, ideally to a center specializing in stroke care. The HINTS examination can be utilized to differentiate between these two conditions and may be performed by a primary care physician.

The HINTS examination comprises three components:

1. Head impulse test in the horizontal plane (h-HIT).

2. Assessment of whether the direction of nystagmus remains consistent regardless of the direction of gaze.

3. Assessment for skew deviation (oblique ocular misalignment) conducted during the initial gaze examination. Skew deviation refers to a vertical misalignment of the eyes when positioned in the primary gaze.

In the h-HIT, it is recommended that the subject maintain fixation on a designated point situated at least 0.5 meters directly in front of them. This point may be represented by the tip of the examiner's nose. Concurrently, the examiner should securely stabilize the patient's head with both hands on either side. Subsequently, the examiner will swiftly rotate the subject's head approximately 20 degrees to one side. After returning the head to the neutral position, the examiner will then turn the subject's head in the opposite direction. Under normal peripheral vestibular function, the eyes remain stable during these head movements. Conversely, in the presence of vestibular dysfunction—particularly when the head is turned toward the side of the affected vestibular organ—the eyes initially move in the same direction as the head, followed by a rapid corrective movement back toward the fixation point. These rapid corrective eye movements are referred to as saccades. In the context of the h-HIT, only those saccades that occur after the head movement (post-saccades) are observable without specialized equipment. The detection of saccades during the h-HIT indicates the presence of peripheral vestibular impairment (**Figure 3**).

In the assessment that evaluates whether the direction of nystagmus remains consistent regardless of gaze direction, it is recommended that the patient with nystagmus focus on a finger positioned approximately 30 cm in front of their eyes. The examiner should then move the finger laterally, first to one side and then to the other. In cases of peripheral damage, the intensity of nystagmus will increase when the patient gazes in the direction of the fast phase and will decrease when looking toward the slow phase. Importantly, the direction of the nystagmus will remain unchanged irrespective of the gaze direction. Conversely, any alteration in the direction of nystagmus accompanying a change in gaze direction suggests the presence of central damage (**Figure 4**).

The skew deviation assessment is conducted by alternately covering and uncovering the patient's eyes. Following the uncovering of an eye, the presence of disjunctive vertical eye movements—specifically, one eye drifting downward while the other

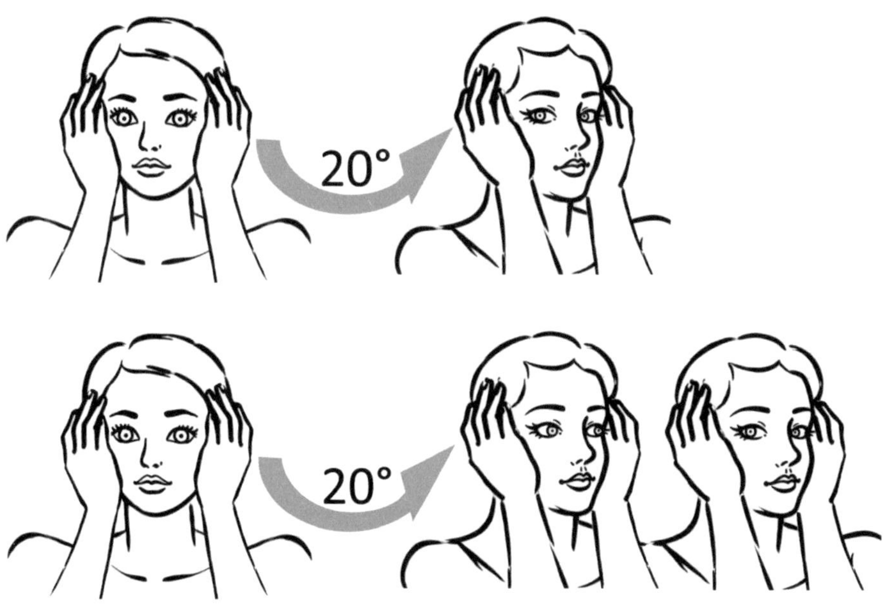

Figure 3.
Head impulse test in the horizontal plane (h-HIT).

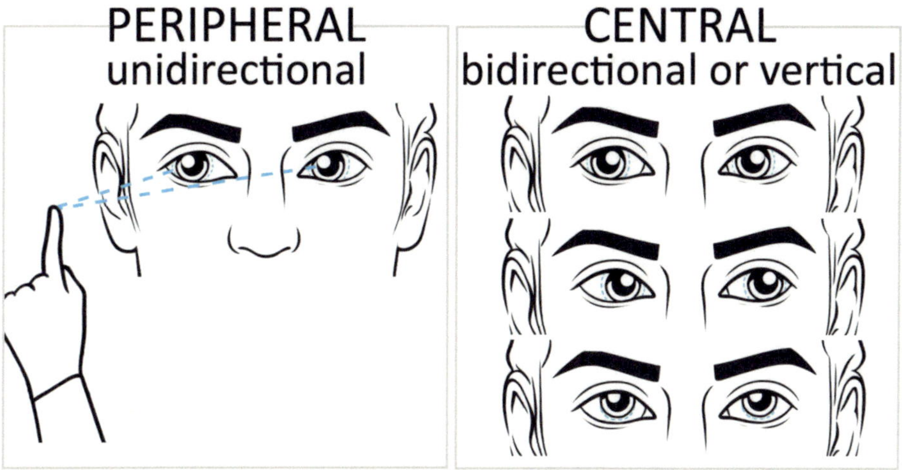

Figure 4.
Evaluation of whether the direction of nystagmus remains consistent across different gaze positions.

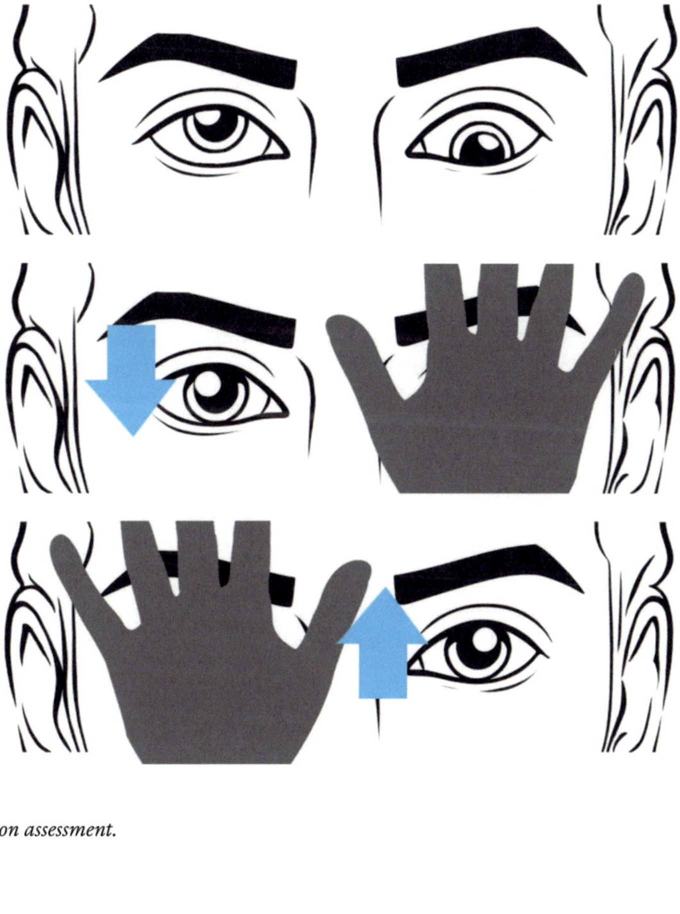

Figure 5.
The skew deviation assessment.

drifts upward—suggests a lesion within the central nervous system. Pathological skew deviations are most characteristic of brainstem strokes (**Figure 5**) [36].

Kattah et al. report that the HINTS examination demonstrates greater sensitivity and specificity in distinguishing vestibular neuritis from strokes involving the vertebrobasilar territory within the first 72 hours of symptom onset compared to diffusion-weighted MRI (DWI MRI) [37].

7. Conclusions

This comprehensive review underscores the complexity and high prevalence of vestibular disorders encountered in primary care settings, highlighting the critical importance of accurate diagnosis and prompt management. Symptoms such as vertigo, dizziness, and balance disturbances are common and significantly impair patients' quality of life, particularly among aging populations. These presentations often pose diagnostic challenges due to their multifactorial etiology, which encompasses peripheral, central, systemic, and psychological factors.

The review emphasizes the necessity for primary care physicians to differentiate benign vestibular conditions—such as benign paroxysmal positional vertigo (BPPV), vestibular migraine, vestibular neuritis, and Ménière's disease—from more serious central or systemic neurological pathologies. Essential clinical assessments include comprehensive history-taking, physical examination, and bedside tests such as the Romberg and Fukuda Unterberger maneuvers. The identification of characteristic vestibular nystagmus patterns and the application of the Head-Impulse, Nystagmus, Test of Skew (HINTS) exam are pivotal in distinguishing peripheral vestibular deficits from central causes like stroke, thereby facilitating timely urgent interventions.

Furthermore, recognizing red flags—such as new neurological deficits or signs indicative of cerebrovascular events—is vital for determining the need for urgent hospital referral. Appropriately directing patients to specialists, including otolaryngologists, neurologists, or rehabilitation therapists, based on clinical findings, ensures comprehensive and targeted care.

In summary, effective management of vestibular symptoms requires a thorough understanding of their clinical presentation, judicious use of bedside diagnostic tools, vigilant identification of red flags, and timely referral. These strategies are essential to optimize patient outcomes, reduce fall risk, prevent injury, and mitigate long-term disability.

Author details

Michalina Piechocka* and Przemysław Śpiewak
Audiofonika – Audiology and Phoniatrics Otpatient Clinic, Bielsko-Biała, Poland

*Address all correspondence to: misiaspiewak@gmail.com

References

[1] Bisdorff A, Von Brevern M, Lempert T, Newman-Toker DE. Classification of vestibular symptoms: Towards an international classification of vestibular disorders. Journal of Vestibular Research. 2009;**19**(1-2):1-13. DOI: 10.3233/VES-2009-0343

[2] Zwergal A, Mantokoudis G, Heg D, et al. What is the current status of primary care in the diagnosis and treatment of patients with vertigo and dizziness in Switzerland? A national survey. Frontiers in Neurology. 2023;**14**:1254080. DOI: 10.3389/fneur.2023.1254080

[3] Chang J, Hwang SY, Park SK, Kim JH, Kim HJ, Chae SW, et al. Prevalence of dizziness and associated factors in South Korea: A cross-sectional survey from 2010 to 2012. Journal of Epidemiology. 2018;**28**:176-184. DOI: 10.2188/jea.JE20160113

[4] Bösner S, Schwarm S, Grevenrath P, et al. Prevalence, aetiologies and prognosis of the symptom dizziness in primary care – A systematic review. BMC Family Practice. 2018;**19**:33. DOI: 10.1186/s12875-017-0695-0

[5] Neuhauser HK. The epidemiology of dizziness and vertigo. Handbook of Clinical Neurology. 2016;**137**:67-82. DOI: 10.1016/B978-0-444-63437-5.00005-4

[6] Wojtczak R, Narożny W, Kuczkowski J, et al. Epidemiology of dizziness in northern Poland – The first polish neurootologic survey of the general population. Annals of Agricultural and Environmental Medicine. 2017;**24**:502-506. DOI: 10.5604/12321966.1228401

[7] Kerber KA, Callaghan BC, Telian SA, Meurer WJ, Skolarus LE, Carender W, et al. Dizziness symptom type prevalence and overlap: A US nationally representative survey. The American Journal of Medicine. 2017;**130**:e1461-e1465. DOI: 10.1016/j.amjmed.2017.05.048

[8] Murdin L, Schilder AGM. Epidemiology of balance symptoms and disorders in the community: A systematic review. Otology & Neurotology. 2015;**36**(3):38. DOI: 10.1097/MAO.0000000000000691

[9] Kammerlind AS, Peolsson A, Johansson MM. Dizziness in older persons at high risk of future hospitalization: Prevalence, differences between those with and without dizziness, and effect of a proactive primary care intervention. BMC Geriatrics. 2022;**22**(1):315. DOI: 10.1186/s12877-022-02910-1

[10] Lindell E, Kollen L, Johansson M, Karlsson T, Ryden L, Fassberg MM, et al. Dizziness and health-related quality of life among older adults in an urban population: A cross-sectional study. Health and Quality of Life Outcomes. 2021;**19**:231. DOI: 10.1186/s12955-021-01864-z

[11] Bisdorff A, Bosser G, Gueguen R, Perrin P. The epidemiology of vertigo, dizziness, and unsteadiness and its links to co-morbidities. Frontiers in Neurology. 2013;**4**:29. DOI: 10.3389/fneur.2013.00029

[12] Neuhauser HK, Radtke A, Von Brevern M, Lezius F, Feldmann M, Lempert T. Burden of dizziness and vertigo in the community. Archives of Internal Medicine. 2008;**168**:2118-2124. DOI: 10.1001/archinte.168.19.2118

[13] Bronstein AM, Golding JF, Gresty MA, et al. The social impact of dizziness in London and Siena. Journal of Neurology. 2010;**257**(2):183-190. DOI: 10.1007/s00415-009-5287-z

[14] De Moraes SA, Soares WJ, Ferriolli E, Perracini MR. Prevalence and correlates of dizziness in community-dwelling older people: A cross sectional population based study. BMC Geriatrics. 2013;**13**:4. DOI: 10.1186/1471-2318-13-4

[15] Van de Berg R, Murdin L, Whitney SL, Holmberg J, Bisdorff A. Curriculum for vestibular medicine (VestMed) proposed by the Bárány society. The concept of vestibular medicine and the framework defining the knowledge, skills and attitudes needed for proficiency in vestibular medicine. Journal of Vestibular Research. 2022;**32**(2):89-98. DOI: 10.3233/VES-210095

[16] Śpiewak M, Śpiewak P, Piechocki M, et al. Vestibulometry, the registration of responses to stimulation of the vestibular organ with stimuli of different frequencies. Otolaryngologia Polska. 2024;**78**(6):20-26. DOI: 10.5604/01.3001.0054.7085

[17] Ganz JA, Sinks BC, Goebel JA. The vertigo case history. In: Jacobson G, Shepard N, editors. Balance Function Assessment and Management. San Diego: Plural Publishing; 2021. pp. 125-136

[18] Woroń J, Jurkiewicz D, Rapiejko P, Lorkowska-Zawicka P, Tymiński R, Wordliczek J. Drug-induced diseases in otolaryngology–causes, clinical signs, treatment. Otolaryngologia Polska. 2021;**75**(2):1-5

[19] Von Brevern M, Bertholon P, Brandt T, Fife T, Imai T, Nuti D, et al. Benign paroxysmal positional vertigo: Diagnostic criteria. Journal of Vestibular Research. 2015;**25**(3-4):105-117. DOI: 10.3233/VES-150553

[20] Strupp M, Lopez-Escamez JA, Kim JS, Straumann D, Jen JC, Carey J, et al. Vestibular paroxysmia: Diagnostic criteria. Journal of Vestibular Research. 2016;**26**(5-6):409-415. DOI: 10.3233/VES-160589

[21] Lopez-Escamez JA, Carey J, Chung WH, Goebel JA, Magnusson M, Mandalà M, et al. Diagnostic criteria for Meniere's disease. Journal of Vestibular Research. 2015;**25**(1):1-7. DOI: 10.3233/VES-150549

[22] Lempert T, Olesen J, Furman J, Waterston J, Seemungal B, Carey J, et al. Vestibular migraine: Diagnostic criteria 1. Journal of Vestibular Research. 2022;**32**(1):1-6. DOI: 10.3233/VES-201644

[23] Strupp M, Bisdorff A, Furman J, Hornibrook J, Jahn K, Maire R, et al. Acute unilateral vestibulopathy/vestibular neuritis: Diagnostic criteria. Journal of Vestibular Research. 2022;**32**(5):389-406. DOI: 10.3233/VES-220201

[24] Cha YH, Baloh RW, Cho C, Magnusson M, Song JJ, Strupp M, et al. Mal de débarquement syndrome diagnostic criteria: Consensus document of the classification Committee of the Bárány Society. Journal of Vestibular Research. 2020;**30**(5):285-293. DOI: 10.3233/VES-200714

[25] Staab JP, Eckhardt-Henn A, Horii A, Jacob R, Strupp M, Brandt T, et al. Diagnostic criteria for persistent postural-perceptual dizziness (PPPD): Consensus document of the committee for the classification of vestibular disorders of the Bárány society. Journal of Vestibular Research. 2017;**27**(4):191-208. DOI: 10.3233/VES-170622

[26] Verriello L, Pauletto G, Nilo A, Lonigro I, Betto E, Valente M, et al. Epilepsy and episodic ataxia type 2: Family study and review of the literature. Journal of Neurology. 2021;**268**(11):4296-4302. DOI: 10.1007/s00415-021-10555-0

[27] Forbes J, Munakomi S, Cronovich HA. Romberg Test. In: StatPearls [Internet]. Treasure Island. FL: StatPearls Publishing; 2025

[28] Unterberger S. Neue objektiv registrierbare Vestibularis-Körperdrehreaktion, erhalten durch Treten auf der Stelle Der Tretversuch. Archiv für Ohren-, Nasen- und Kehlkopfheilkunde. 1938;**145**:273-282. DOI: 10.1007/BF01583067

[29] Fukuda T. The stepping test: Two phases of the labyrinthine reflex. Acta Oto-Laryngologica. 1959;**50**:95-108. DOI: 10.3109/00016485909129172

[30] Hemm S, Baumann D, Duarte da Costa V, Tarnutzer AA. Test-re-test reliability and dynamics of the Fukuda-Unterberger stepping test. Frontiers in Neurology. 2023;**14**:1128760. DOI: 10.3389/fneur.2023.1128760

[31] Cohen HS, Sangi-Haghpeykar H, Ricci NA, Kampangkaew J, Williamson RA. Utility of stepping, walking, and head impulses for screening patients for vestibular impairments. Otolaryngology and Head and Neck Surgery. 2014;**151**:131-136. DOI: 10.1177/0194599814527724

[32] Honaker JA, Shepard NT. Performance of Fukuda stepping test as a function of the severity of caloric weakness in chronic dizzy patients. Journal of the American Academy of Audiology. 2012;**23**:616-622. DOI: 10.3766/jaaa.23.8.6

[33] Tarnutzer AA, Duarte Da Costa V, Baumann D, Hemm S. Heading direction is significantly biased by preceding whole-body roll-orientation while lying. Frontiers in Neurology. 2022;**13**:868144. DOI: 10.3389/fneur.2022.868144

[34] Eggers S. Practical anatomy and physiology of the ocular motor system. In: Jacobson G, Shepard N, editors. Balance Function Assessment and Management. San Diego: Plural Publishing; 2021. pp. 43-68

[35] Strupp ML, Straumann D, Helmchen C. Nystagmus: Diagnosis, topographic anatomical localization and therapy. Klinische Monatsblätter für Augenheilkunde. 2021;**238**(11):1186-1195. DOI: 10.1055/a-1525-0030

[36] Kattah JC. Use of HINTS in the acute vestibular syndrome. An overview. Stroke and Vascular Neurology. 2018;**3**(4):190-196. DOI: 10.1136/svn-2018-000160

[37] Kattah JC, Talkad AV, Wang DZ, Yu-Hsiang Hsieh D, Newman-Toker DE. HINTS to diagnose stroke in the acute vestibular syndrome: Three-step bedside oculomotor examination more sensitive than early MRI diffusion-weighted imaging. Stroke. 2009;**40**(11):3504-3510. DOI: 10.1161/STROKEAHA.109.551234